# THE ULTIMATE STRESS-RELIEF PLAN FOR WOMEN

STEPHANIE McCLELLAN, M.D.
*and* BETH HAMILTON, M.D.

*with* DIANE REVERAND

Previously published as *So Stressed*

FREE PRESS
New York London Toronto Sydney

Free Press
A Division of Simon & Schuster, Inc.
1230 Avenue of the Americas
New York, NY 10020

First Free Press trade paperback edition May 2011

FREE PRESS and colophon are trademarks of Simon & Schuster, Inc.

For information about special discounts for bulk purchases,
please contact Simon & Schuster Special Sales at
1-866-506-1949 or business@simonandschuster.com.

The Simon & Schuster Speakers Bureau can bring authors to your
live event. For more information or to book an event contact the
Simon & Schuster Speakers Bureau at 1-866-248-3049 or visit
our website at www.simonspeakers.com.

Designed by Julie Schroeder

Manufactured in the United States of America

10  9  8  7  6  5  4  3  2  1

The Library of Congress has cataloged the hardcover edition as follows:

McClellan, Stephanie.
    So stressed : the ultimate stress-relief plan for women /
Stephanie McClellan and Beth Hamilton; with Diane Reverand.
        p. cm.
    Includes bibliographical references and index.
    1. Stress management for women.    I. Hamilton, Beth.
II. Reverand, Diane.    III. Title.
    RA785.M385 2009
    616.9'80082—dc22                                2009036176

ISBN 978-1-4165-9358-4
ISBN 978-1-4165-9359-1 (pbk)
ISBN 978-1-4391-0055-4 (ebook)

Previously published as *So Stressed*.

For our mothers, our sisters, our dear friends, and our patients
For our favorite men
Bob, Michael, Tyler, and Gunnar
SNMCC
Jeff, Jake, and Asher
BH

# CONTENTS

# STANDING IN THE GAP
# (OR WHY WE ARE WRITING THIS BOOK)

As practicing gynecologists, we see the devastating effects of stress on our patients' health and sense of well-being every day. In women of all ages, whether or not they are aware of it, stress disrupts their bodies' intricate balance and creates illness. Without question, stress is at the root of many of the physical problems we treat.

Our decision to write this book crept up on us. Early in our practice of medicine, we recognized that stress was behind many, if not most, health problems. During our years of clinical practice, as we tried to correct the conditions and issues that stress gives rise to, we saw even more clearly the direct link between the stress that our patients experienced and the diseases they developed. As we kept up with the latest research, we read studies that correlated stress with high blood pressure and heart disease, which today is widely known. But we also suspected that stress is less obviously linked to other diseases and disorders, such as chronic pain, weight gain, allergies, diabetes, decreased libido, and autoimmune disorders like rheumatoid arthritis.

Sometimes patients come to us with troubling symptoms that defy diagnosis. We send them for tests and refer them to other specialists if necessary, to help manage their symptoms, but they still may not receive a clear diagnosis. In many cases, their symptoms improve markedly only after they make significant changes in their own lives. For instance, one teenage girl with a domineering mother suffered debilitating pelvic pain for years and even had two surgeries, which gave her little relief. It was not until she left home for college that she became pain free. A brilliant doctor and mother of three developed a tremor in her hands and blinding headaches and feared she was developing Parkinson's disease or multiple sclerosis. When a battery of tests came back negative, she was forced to examine the pace at which she was living her life. After a few simple lifestyle changes that reduced stress, she was back to normal in very little time.

Having seen countless cases like these, we decided to dig deeper to uncover the roots of stress and to understand how it can lead to so many different physical problems. In the process of finding direct links to multiple disorders other than cardiovascular diseases, we changed the way we practice medicine. Having always asked about our patients' lives as well as their health, we had consistently developed a full picture of our patients as whole women and individuals, not just collections of symptoms. Now, in addition, we incorporated recommendations on nutrition, exercise, and restoration techniques in our treatment program—recommendations tailored to suit each patient and her living circumstances. Once we saw the many concrete effects of stress, we could no longer simply accept them as inevitable and inescapable. We were impelled to educate our patients about what we'd discovered in our research and to provide them with new ways to break the stress-illness link, to heal and prevent stress-related problems. **Our aim in writing this book is to give you a greater understanding of how stress works in your body and to recommend effective ways for you to overcome its destructive effects and return to health.**

Some years ago, we refined a minimally invasive "outpatient" hysterectomy procedure performed by laparoscopy. This technique has allowed our patients to recover more quickly than they would from a traditional hysterectomy and allows them to recuperate in the comfort of their homes. Not only is their recovery faster, but their pain is significantly reduced, because their stress and anxiety about the surgical procedure is minimized. This breakthrough in treatment and improved recovery was another significant indication to us of how profoundly stress affects our patients and how reducing their stress improves the quality of their lives.

As a woman, you want to be responsible for your good health. You read magazines and books, turn to the internet with your medical questions, and hear about the latest "miracle cures" on television and radio shows. You are inundated with conflicting advice and misinformation that can overwhelm you, leaving you feeling confused, helpless, and hopeless. Our mission is to help you ask the right questions, so that you better understand your body and its strengths and vulnerabilities. For instance, why do you collapse on vacation and become sick and withdrawn, unable to join in the fun with your partner or family? Or why, as a working mother, are you suddenly depressed and getting high-blood-pressure readings? These setbacks could be the result of chronic stress that affects your body and mind in ways you can learn to predict, block, and manage.

A single theme emerges in our conversations with our patients: **almost every woman we see expresses in varying degrees a sense that her life and health are not as they should be.** Our patients often begin our conversations by saying, "I am so stressed," or, "I've been under a lot of stress lately." They are pressured, rushed, edgy, or totally exhausted. Stress is robbing women of joy and of a sense of purpose in their lives. At our office every day, we see what stress is doing to women—their ashen skin tone, the bags under their eyes, dull, dry hair, sleeping problems, depression, and pain. Some describe such physical symptoms as aching joints or weight gain that they don't realize correlate directly with their stress. Others, particularly women in their forties and fifties, don't even want to admit that stress is getting to them, as if being stressed out were a sign of weakness or failure. As we educate each patient about the many effects that stress has on her particular body and brain, sometimes it feels as if stress is all we ever talk about.

As women and physicians, we are more than sympathetic—we are intimately familiar with the subject. Each of us has a family—five sons between us—and we work long, intense hours, including two days of surgery every week. We could be poster girls for stress if we didn't follow our own advice.

In our practice as medical doctors with a specialty in gynecology (and previously, also obstetrics), we are devoted to delivering the highest-quality health care to our patients. In our practice, in Newport Beach, California, which we call OC Gyn, we treat thousands of women a year, many of whom come from all over the United States and as far away as Asia and Europe. We have developed a reputation for providing clear, scientific explanations to our patients about what causes illness and what creates health. In this way, we act as health advocates for our patients, enabling them to make informed decisions with us about their care.

In *The Ultimate Stress-Relief Plan for Women*, we aim to make the pertinent science of health and illness accessible, answer questions, and recommend solutions.

When we set out to cover the most recent science regarding women and stress, we discovered even more exciting research than we had expected. So many new discoveries are being made every day. We visited or communicated with the world's leading researchers in Germany, Sweden, and New York City's Rockefeller Institute on stress's effects on health. We immersed ourselves in mountains of scientific papers. As we read, talked with experts, and treated our patients, we realized that we are standing in the gap between the brilliant research being done around the world in laboratories today and the actual use of those findings in clinical practice in doctors' offices. Bridging the gap from lab bench to bedside, and now, to a book, we aim to translate groundbreaking science into techniques that help women deal with stress in their daily lives.

In caring for our patients, we have to take into account physical and psychological concerns, hormones and neuroscience, and a host of other factors so that we can create an integrated, comprehensive treatment for their individual health problems. Since many women visit a doctor only to see their gynecologist for their annual exam, we end up being primary-care doctors for many of our patients. We deal one-on-one with women who need our help with a broad range of ailments, and our combined experience of nearly forty years has led us to develop a strong practical, problem-solving approach. We are not doing research in a lab or lecturing at a university. **We deal with real women with real health issues and offer them real solutions every day.**

Besides the gap between lab bench and medical practice, we are standing in another gap as well—the gap that exists between the current health care system and the real needs of women for the best possible individualized care. All physicians face real challenges in trying to deliver that care. Our medical system has little to do with wellness; it is best at caring for people once they are sick. But in order to provide the best possible care, medicine and its practitioners must begin to prevent disease and educate patients about issues that promote disease. Today, when a patient has a number of health problems at the same time, the system treats each illness separately. Our health care system does not consolidate treatment or identify common causes for multiple disorders. This is why you may have had to go to several specialists to find the answers to your health problems—an integrated approach to health does not exist.

Health care for women is especially inadequate. Our health care system tends to patronize or ignore women and has traditionally treated them as second-class citizens. Until recently, medical scientific research had rarely involved women in studies because of the influence of our hormonal cycles on our physiology. Women were excluded from studies that formed the basis of the most common treatments that both men and women receive, including medications, which are prescribed for both sexes in the same doses. This means that a slim woman of five feet four inches often gets the same heart or blood-pressure medication as a man who has eight inches of height and a hundred pounds over her. No wonder the American Heart Association has established a new field of study focusing on heart disease in women. Scientists have only recently learned how different cardiovascular disease is for women than for men; and that's only one of the major fields to have recent breakthroughs.

During our research for this book, however, we were pleased to discover that women are now included more often in current studies. The tide is turning because women control more money, which increases our power and forces service providers to listen to us, to become more accountable, and to provide better health care. Until the Women's Health Initiative, in 2001, no significant, controlled, double-blind study had been performed on the multisystem effects of hormone therapy, even though it had been commonly prescribed for more than fifty years. Historically, more money was spent marketing health care to women than to supporting substantial medical research on women's health, because women make the medical choices in most families, selecting doctors, hospitals, and sometimes insurance carriers. In other words, **the medical establishment would rather appeal to your buying power than your health needs.**

We believe that women deserve the attention of the health care community as individuals and as the foundation of families. Strong, healthy women make strong, healthy societies.

The life span of both men and women has changed dramatically in the last hundred years, but a more significant change has occurred in the way people live. Women in particular are under greater stress than ever as we balance many roles, including being loving wives and mothers, fostering a rich family life, running households, working outside the home and running companies, engaging in community service and activities, and often caring for elderly parents living near or far. **Our bodies are unable to handle the insidious effects of this constant stress because our biology has not changed to accommodate the new demands of our multiple roles.** At the same time, modern life has reduced the everyday social support that is one of our basic human needs—as well as a preventer and healer of stress. The latest advances in communications have all made us more available to anyone at any time, disturbing our peace and increasingly isolating us.

We want to help you realize how stress affects every cell of your body and the way your mind experiences the world and translates its feelings to your body, so that you can take steps to stay healthy or get healthy. We want you to be able to identify how you typically respond to stress, so we've described four basic stress types to help you determine what type you are. We alert you to the danger signs that arise when stress becomes destructive and provide you with a program for reducing stress based on your specific type.

As we make recommendations to help you get healthy and reduce the stress in your life, we also reveal the amazing interactions of your body's intricate inner systems. Our researching this book has made us even more awestruck by the female body's strength, beauty, and resilience, and we want to communicate the wonder we feel at the complex systems that run our bodies and serve us so brilliantly. We hope that our reports on the latest scientific research on women and stress will give you new insights into your own strengths and resilience. We want to help you take control of your reaction to the enormous stress you face today, so that you can feel your best physically, mentally, and emotionally.

—Stephanie McClellan, MD, and Beth Hamilton, MD

INTRODUCTION

# WHY ARE WOMEN
# SO STRESSED?

With all that is going on in the world, it's no wonder that we are experiencing a stress epidemic. It's time to learn about the toll that stress
takes on your well-being. Research has shown that the effects of stress
are more extreme for women than for men: women release more of
the chemical triggers for stress, and these hormones remain longer in
a woman's body than a man's. Female hormones directly influence
your response to stress. Women also appear to be more susceptible
to the physical symptoms of stress due to gender differences in brain
processing, which we will explain later. As a result of these biological
differences, women tend to be more sensitive to stress, and the stress
response lasts longer in the female body than in the male.

## MULTITASKING YOUR WAY TO EXHAUSTION

Even though women are biologically equipped to do many things at
once, we never seem to have enough time to do all that we need to
do. Our brains are actually hardwired to enable us to multitask, so,
because we're good at it, we push the envelope and try to do more,
thinking we can handle just one more thing. But whenever we try to
do too much—and what woman doesn't—we create a nagging sense
of urgency and the feeling that we will never catch up. We race from

one activity or chore to another, stretching ourselves to the limit, rarely taking time to relax. Women are also conditioned to be responsive to others' well-being and to try to please. This nurturing tendency makes us susceptible to higher stress levels when we take on too much and find ourselves on overload.

Most women have numerous roles and are expected to assume all or some of the following:

Wife

Mother

Daughter

Health care provider for a parent

Sister

Friend

Employee

Household manager

Cook/nutritionist

Personal shopper

Crisis manager

Cheerleader

Social director

Housekeeper

Chauffeur

Tutor

Mediator

Party planner

Life coach

Volunteer

Interior decorator

Hair stylist

Dog walker and trainer

Nurse

Laundress

Fitness and nutrition advocate

Financial manager/bill payer

Gardener

Some believe that the greatest contributor to the epidemic of stress among women now is that they are working outside the home in record numbers. At the turn of the twentieth century, only 12 percent of women were paid a salary for their work; today, we comprise 46 percent of the workforce. Seventy percent of mothers with children under the age of eighteen now work. Either raising children or working requires much more than half our attention, on top of which working women still have primary responsibility for child care and household chores. **A worldwide survey of women between the ages of thirteen and sixty-five found that women who work full-time and have children under the age of thirteen report the greatest stress.**

Working mothers can become stressed because they feel guilty for leaving their children. Yet women who choose to stay home to raise their children often feel isolated and stressed because they are not contributing financially. Their husbands often have to work long hours as the sole income earner, which can also become a source of friction. And married women who have not worked outside the home or who are widowed or lose their financial security after a divorce have multiple financial stresses and usually a marked decline in their quality of life.

**A recent American Psychological Association Poll (2007) found that 48 percent of Americans say they are more stressed now than they were five years ago.** Money and work top the list of what 75 percent of Americans worry about, a big leap from 59 percent two years earlier. And that poll was taken before the global financial crisis of fall 2008. The impact of this constant stress is staggering:

- Forty-four percent of all adults suffer adverse health effects from stress.
- Ninety-five percent of all office visits to physicians are for stress-related ailments.
- Stress is linked to the six leading causes of death: heart disease, cancer, lung ailments, accidents, liver disease, and suicide.

**Two kinds of stresses are at work on all of us every day—chronic and acute.** Chronic stress is long-term, unrelenting, and seemingly inescapable; it wears down your body, mind, and spirit. Acute stresses—life's traumatic events and most-challenging situations—can also send your stress levels off the charts.

## THE TWO BASIC RESPONSES TO CHRONIC STRESS

After caring for thousands of patients at OC Gyn, we have seen that women have two basic responses to stress—hyperactive and hypoactive. With a hyperactive stress response, you're frantically trying to wrestle with everything that's troubling you at once; a hypoactive stress response is when you are too drained to deal with even the most-pressing problems. Of course, the line between hyperactive and hypoactive is a dynamic one, and patients' symptoms can vary in different situations; often, they move somewhere along the scale between the two. Wherever you are on the continuum of hyperactive stress response or hypoactive stress response, you're not feeling well.

**The two basic stress responses break down into four types of stress-caused imbalance that can vary in degree from mild to extreme.** Each type displays its own symptoms and each has particular tendencies to develop certain diseases. Specific diet, exercise, and relaxation techniques create physiological effects that bring the body closer to balance. The point from which you start is what matters. Different imbalances respond to type-specific relaxation techniques and diet and exercise tailored to the individual.

Today, most people expect and sometimes demand that doctors help them by prescribing a pill that will make them feel better. But at OC Gyn, we do not pull out the prescription pad quite so readily. We prefer to educate our patients about the consequences of long-term stress and then to develop individualized stress-relief programs that address their imbalance.

The four type-specific programs for diffusing stress that we've devised are far more powerful than any pill available, and their side effects are beneficial. By learning how to defuse stress in a way that works for you, you can take control of your health and prevent more serious diseases from developing. If you already have an illness, reducing stress will help your body deal with the illness and help you heal.

First, we tell you what stress looks like, its outward signs, and give you a sense of how it affects your behavior, emotions, and health. In chapter 2, "The Psychology of Stress," we explore how your perceptions of stress and certain patterns of thinking often evoke the stress response. Then, in chapter 3, we describe "the anatomy of stress" and how your body is wired to respond. We help you determine which of the four types of stress response is your type and show you how to alleviate your stress using healthy, sustainable techniques.

We'll examine the negative effects of stress, including the complaints we hear most often and the conditions we see—weight gain, fatigue, chronic pain, cardiovascular disease, and metabolic syndrome, a group of risk factors that include weight gain around the abdomen, high cholesterol, high blood pressure, and a high inflammatory response. We'll show you how to combat these and more in part 2, "The Stress-Detox Programs," in which we describe the anatomy of relaxation, methods for changing your psychological and physiological response to potentially stressful situations, with specific recommendations about diet, exercise, and relaxation techniques to help you avoid the negative effects of stress or to reverse any harm that has already been done. We provide you with a Stress Program Log that you can use to record your commitment and progress in these areas. We also suggest you keep a Stress Journal as you read through the book to keep track of the information that relates specifically to you. With the simple, scientifically based methods explained in "The Stress Detox Programs," you will be able to deal effectively with the way your body responds to stress.

Once you understand what out-of-control stress does to you, we hope that you will be inspired to trust in your own power to withstand it and to make choices in your life that will promote your good health, resilience, and pleasure.

# PART ONE

# IDENTIFY
# YOUR
# STRESS TYPE

# CHAPTER ONE

# HOW STRESS LOOKS

S ally, a twenty-five-year-old mother of a young son, sat rigidly on the examining table, looking thin and frail. Her eyes were puffy, her skin dull. She had made an appointment to see Stephanie again because her vaginal pain and discharge, which had been occurring for several months, had not responded to various treatments. She was terrified, convinced that she had terminal cancer.

Her examination revealed swelling and redness. Under the microscope, the sample showed huge numbers of inflammatory cells without obvious offending bacteria or yeast. Sally fit a diagnosis of desquamitive inflammatory vaginitis, which stems from an overactive immune system. Her immune system was attacking the cells of her vagina as if they were foreign, leading to outright pain, excessive vaginal secretions, and difficulty having intercourse. Sally did not appear relieved when Stephanie assured her that there was a treatment that would probably resolve her condition completely. She was still convinced that she had a serious illness, because she felt miserable and had been getting worse.

Our clinical experience at OC Gyn has shown that this is a stress-related condition, but Sally had not made a connection between any stress she was experiencing and her persistent physical problem. When Stephanie asked Sally directly if she was experiencing more stress than usual, Sally cracked and began to cry. She confided that her son was defiant and extremely demanding. Her husband worked long hours in hopes of moving up at his job and was never home. She had no help, because her husband felt it was an unnecessary expense and they were saving for a new home with room for more children. No family members lived nearby to give her a hand; she had to do it all alone and felt isolated. By the time her husband came home, she was exhausted and irritable. She didn't mean to be difficult, especially since he was working so hard, but all they seemed to do was bicker.

Sally's stress had been so bottled up within her that she simply couldn't stop crying now that she was admitting how hard things were for her. Stephanie listened, let her vent, and consoled her as best she could. When Sally calmed down, they discussed a treatment plan for her vaginal condition, and Stephanie explained that she would not get better until she addressed her stress level. Stephanie explained how important it was, not so much because Sally was physically uncomfortable but because the stress was clearly affecting her immune function and could lead to more serious health consequences. Stephanie suggested that Sally seek professional therapy and also find some time for herself.

At Sally's return visit a few weeks later, her physical condition had improved, because she had been compliant about taking her medication, but she had not made any changes to affect the quality of her life. She broke down crying again, still convinced that she had a life-threatening illness. Stephanie explained once more that the seriousness of her condition involved her inordinate stress and advised Sally that unless she did something to relieve her stress, she really could develop a life-threatening condition.

At her next visit, a month later, Sally smiled when Stephanie walked into the room—things obviously had changed. She was full of energy. Her skin was bright and smooth, her hair brushed and groomed. The symptoms that had brought her to the office initially were gone. Sally had talked with her husband about Stephanie's advice for reducing her extreme stress levels, and he had agreed to hire a babysitter a few times a week to give her some relief. She was taking a spin class and had joined a mothers' group at the community center. She was back to being her vivacious self.

Susan, thirty-two, is all too aware of how stress is affecting her, because her chronic bladder infections tend to flare up when she is under stress. During her last visit to our offices, she talked to Beth about the correlation between the infections and the amount of pressure in her life. She had a lot going on: she had been caring for her mother, who was recovering from a mastectomy; she had a new man in her life; and she had moved her household. That's three of life's major stressors. She had been so busy with her mother that she hadn't even had time to unpack and settle into her new place and was still living out of cartons.

Stress can impair your immune system, which makes it hard for the body to fight off infections. Since Beth had treated Susan for other chronic urinary-tract infections, she suggested that Susan change her diet to incorporate probiotics, which are dietary supplements or foods that resemble the beneficial microorganisms found in your digestive system. Then, Beth made recommendations about how Susan could reduce her stress, encouraging her to take the time to unpack and settle into her new home. With Susan's input, she designed a program of exercise and nutrition. She also advised her to take breaks and listen to music whenever dealing with her mother's illness became overwhelming. Susan was happy to know that she had been correct about the root of her problem and was motivated to make these changes in her life to improve her health.

## YOUR RESPONSE TO STRESS IS UNIQUE

Stress looks different on different people. **Your reaction to stress is multifaceted and is shaped by your psychology, physiology, genetic makeup, and environment.** Every woman's response to stress is unique, so it stands to reason that each woman requires individual ways to manage her stress.

### Factors That Shape a Stress Response
- Age
- Health status
- Type of stressor
- Duration of exposure
- Genetics
- Early childhood experience
- Nutritional status
- Alcohol, drugs, some medications
- Social support
- Beliefs

## WHAT DOCTORS SEE

In our practice, we have become so sensitive to the consequences of stress that we recognize a wide range of telltale signs that indicate a patient is having difficulty coping with the pressures in her life. Women who are affected by stress can be thin or obese. Their posture can be rigid or slumped. They can be vigilant and anxious or subdued and passive. Many are tremulous. As we describe the many other manifestations of stress, you will recognize some of these traits in yourself.

Our patients have varied complaints, but we hear a handful repeatedly: hair loss, losing skin tone, not seeing results from exercise routines, and accumulation of fat around the middle. All these physical changes are a direct result of chronic stress.

## STRESS AND YOUR SKIN

Your skin, the largest organ of your body, reflects your physical and mental health fairly directly. Stress causes eczema, hives, rosacea, psoriasis, alopecia, and vitiligo. There is also a correlation between stress and acne. In fact, there is such a strong connection between the brain and the skin that scientists have named a field of study "psychodermatology."

When stress disturbs the body's homeostasis, or balance, your hormones can malfunction, impairing the rejuvenation of your skin. Skin is always in a process of renewal, which takes twenty-eight days when you are young but slows down as you age. Emotional stress retards cell renewal, destroys collagen fibers in the skin, and breaks down elastin. This means sags and wrinkles. Evidence also suggests that stress causes the barrier protection of the skin to break down, affecting skin hydration and its normal immune function. This breakdown is part of the reason why we often get sick during times of stress.

## STRESS AND YOUR HAIR

Unrelenting stress may result in the thinning and dulling of your hair. Many of our patients who are under chronic stress complain of hair loss. They are troubled by the amount of hair they find in the shower after they wash their hair. Fortunately, stress-related hair thinning will often stop when your stress is resolved or when you learn how to manage it.

In extreme cases, stress can cause significant hair loss in two different ways. It can cause hair to stop growing, a condition called telogen effluvium; this is when some hair follicles go into a resting phase and fall out two to three months later. Usually, the hair grows back within six to nine months. The second condition is known as alopecia, a more inflammatory response. With this condition, hair follicles are attacked by immune cells. This leads to hair loss in patches or on the entire scalp. Alleviating your stress will help these conditions, too.

## STRESS MAKES YOU OLDER

Stress can actually speed up the aging process by harming DNA. Elissa Epel, a psychologist, and Elizabeth Blackburn, a Nobel laureate in cellular biology, discovered this in a landmark research study at the University of California at San Francisco. The study compared thirty-nine healthy mothers who care for a chronically ill child with nineteen women raising a healthy child. They chose to work with mothers of young children because mothers experience chronic stress at a young age; full-time caregivers tend to have little time for themselves and make huge personal sacrifices.

The study had two levels of assessment: physiological and psychological. With a blood test of white cells, they were able to measure damage to DNA, specifically the most fragile part of the chromosome, called the telomere. Telomeres are the protective caps at the ends of chromosomes. The telomeres are instrumental in determining the health and life span of cells. Dr. Blackburn compares them to the tips of shoelaces: if you lose the tips of your shoelaces, they start to fray. The telomeres protect DNA and promote genetic stability in the same way, by preventing the DNA strands from unraveling.

The enzyme telomerase restores the length of the telomeres when they get worn and replenishes a portion of the telomeres, allowing the cell to repair itself. As we get older, telomerase production lessens, and consequently our bodies age. As more cells die, the visible effects of aging—diminished eyesight and hearing, wrinkled skin, and loss of muscle—become apparent.

The findings of this study show that the longer the mothers had been caring for their chronically ill child, the lower their telomerase-repair activity and the worse the state of their DNA. **The cells of the high-stress women appeared to be nine to seventeen years older than the cells of the lower-stressed women.**

In the psychological assessment, the mothers took a written test to measure their perception of the intensity of stress in their lives. Again, the study found that those **women with higher perceived stress had greater cell aging.** Both groups of mothers showed the same relationship between perceived stress and damaged DNA, but the mothers who coped well under stress, as their psychological assessments revealed, who didn't let it get to them, did not suffer the same level of damage to their telomeres.

Though the stress-and-aging study proved that the perception of stress can affect your body on a cellular level, you may not be aware of these effects, or you may have symptoms without a physiological cause. We call this the mind-body disconnect—when a patient has a stress-related disorder even though she does not report feeling stressed or feels that stress is making her sick when there is no evidence of illness in her body.

The mind-body disconnect, also known as "missing covariance," complicates the diagnosis and management of chronic stress. The external signs of stress can appear different from person to person, so try to be aware of any changes in the way you feel and behave. Stress can creep up on you so that you start making accommodations for it—you stop going to the gym as often because of work deadlines; you start drinking more coffee during the day and a couple of glasses of wine in the evening because you can't get to sleep and don't wake up refreshed; you grab fast food instead of a salad between appointments for yourself or your kids. Soon your stress has mounted and become so unrelenting that it takes a profound toll on your body, unless you take steps to defuse your physical and mental response to it. We will help you develop your awareness of when stress is wearing you down and how your body lets you know that's happening with symptoms such as changes in your skin, hair, weight, and mood. We'll give you the tools to stop the destructive effects before your health is damaged.

This following list of symptoms is not complete, but it should give you an idea of the kinds of signs you should look for.

### The Warning Signs and Symptoms of High Stress

- Nervousness or anxiety
- Sadness or depression
- Anger
- Fatigue
- Sleep disorders
- Lack of interest, motivation, or energy
- Inability to concentrate
- Headaches
- Muscle tension, especially in the neck and shoulders
- Upset stomach, bloating, appetite changes
- Dizziness or faintness
- Tightness in chest
- Reduced sexual desire
- Skin problems such as rashes, acne, or hives
- Aches and pain
- Menstrual irregularity
- Constipation or diarrhea
- Hair loss or dullness

If you've ever had any of these symptoms, consider starting a journal. If you have any of these symptoms regularly, make a note of that as well. If you can link them to events or pressures in your life, like deadlines at work or disagreements with your partner or spouse, note that, too. Observing how you feel and behave when you are stressed will help you to identify your stress type, which we will discuss in chapter 4, "Identify Your Type: The Four Stress-Response Patterns."

### The Consequences of Long-term Stress for Women

- Women are more likely than men to report stress (51 percent as opposed to 43 percent, respectively) and report a wider range of stressors, including time constraints, the expectations of others, marital relationships, children, and family health.
- Women are 2.7 times more likely than men to develop autoimmune diseases, which are stress-related conditions, including type 1 diabetes, multiple sclerosis, lupus, rheumatoid arthritis, thyroid disorders, and inflammatory bowel disease.
- Stress-induced heart disease is the number-one killer of women, but only 13 percent of women consider heart disease a health threat.
- Sixty-four percent of women who die suddenly of heart disease had no previous symptoms.
- Stroke kills more women than men; women represent 61 percent of stroke deaths.
- Nearly one-third of women ages eighteen to fifty-nine suffer from a loss of interest in sex.
- Women have a higher prevalence of pain than men and suffer more musculoskeletal pain than men in older age.
- Stressful events, including loss of a loved one, are linked to an increase of breast cancer in women within two years of the event.
- Women with a diagnosis of breast cancer who consider themselves highly stressed are more likely to have a recurrence.

Chronic stress will make you sick. The good news is that you can manage and even change your response to the pressures in your life. When you do, you will look better, feel better, slow the aging process, and lower your risk for disease.

The next chapter will give you an understanding of how your thoughts, emotions, and perceptions shape your stress response.

CHAPTER TWO

# THE PSYCHOLOGY OF STRESS

Though we are not psychologists, we have found that when our patients understand the relationship between stress and emotions, they are better able to find methods to stop a stress response before it happens. Your emotions can set off a powerful physical response that disrupts the balance of many systems in your body. The fact is that the way you interpret events and the emotions that your assessments produce are at the core of your stress response. You have to decide that something is stressful in order for it to feel and be stressful for you. Habitual patterns of thinking and negative, judgmental self-talk—that little voice inside you that comments on who you are, what you do, and everything around you—are responsible for much of the stress in your life. As we advise our patients, after you learn to recognize your automatic thoughts and feelings, you can learn to change them, which will go a long way toward managing your stress.

In this chapter we will give you a crash course in psychology that you'll be able to apply immediately to your life. You'll learn about some simple theories that provide brilliant insights on how your perceptions of the world can create stress for you. For instance, one woman is excited and honored to have been asked to make a presentation at a conference, while another facing the same opportunity is paralyzed

—— 13 ——

with terror at the thought. One woman waits patiently in the waiting room when her doctors are running behind schedule, using the time to thumb through a magazine, while another fumes, looks at her watch, and thinks of all the things she has to do. The main difference between these women's experiences is how they perceive their situation.

No matter what your stress type, understanding how your mind contributes to generating stress will help you deal with external and internal pressures in a healthier way. We provide you with a technique to examine what you are thinking and feeling in a way that will take the sting from your negative emotions and stressful thought patterns, enabling you to change your response.

Psychologists today divide the functions of the mind into cognition, motivation, and emotion. Studies have confirmed that our mind, emotions, and perceptions of stress are elaborately intertwined. **Your interpretation of a situation and the meaning you attach to the source of stress are responsible for the degree and intensity of your response.** Your senses are bombarded by countless things going on around you. You take in so much that your responses are rapid and often automatic, because your survival depends on your knowing whether a situation is dangerous or not. Your mind never stops screening your experiences to determine whether they are harmful, threatening, challenging, or helpful. Richard S. Lazarus, one of the leaders in psychological-stress research, taught that stress is not found in the situation or in the person but is a product of a transaction between the two. He calls this dynamic the transactional stress theory. The idea is that it takes both a stressful circumstance and a vulnerable person to produce a stress reaction.

Think about that for a second. Not all stress is negative and damaging. Stress is not necessarily a bad thing. In fact, perceiving and reacting to stress is essential for your survival. Some exciting stress can be stimulating and challenge you to accomplish great things. You need a certain amount of stress in order to live and perform well. Stress can motivate you, make you alert and productive, and give you vitality. In acute situations, stress puts you at your sharpest. Acute stress can improve memory, hand-eye coordination, and even strength to deal with exceptional situations. Stress can make swimmers swim faster, surgeons more precise, speakers more engaging, and turn mothers into superheroes when their children are in danger.

When you feel you can handle a challenge, stress can promote a feeling of accomplishment. Responding to stressors in an appropriate way is instrumental in performing tasks well and also fundamental to your sense of well-being. But it is difficult to have rewarding and sometimes even functional social interactions if you are always stressed.

**The way you perceive a particular situation determines whether or not it is stressful for you.** Every day, people cope differently with stress in the same context. Although objective reality is not intrinsically stressful, almost all situations have the potential to be so; the way you perceive them determines whether you're the woman with the magazine or the woman fuming in the waiting room. A stressed response—your emotional, behavioral, and physical reactions—results from a mental judgment you've made, whether you've judged an event to be a threat or whether you think you can cope with it.

Your perception of a situation is based on your beliefs, assumptions, values, and conditioning; in the broadest sense, **your response to stress is a product of your past experience, genetic predisposition, personality, lifestyle, and culture.** It's not a straightforward cause-and-effect process, since so many complex, interacting factors are involved, which is why experiencing stress is unique to each person.

## WHAT MAKES YOU DIFFERENT

All of your past experiences influence your thought processes and perception: your health, the quality of your relationships, your responsibilities, support systems, the successes, disappointments, shake-ups,

THE ULTIMATE STRESS-RELIEF PLAN FOR WOMEN — 16

changes, and ordeals that make up your life. These all combine to fuel the stress you feel in different situations and shape how you respond. Sometimes you develop your coping strategies through trial and error: when you find a way of dealing with a problem that works, you tend to repeat it. The problem, though, is that, eventually, you may be repeating a method that is no longer effective. Many people do this, believing that a quick response is preferable to a new response that may take longer to learn. In the long run, the same old solutions generally stop working—at which point they give you more stress, not less.

**The way you respond to stress is influenced by factors determined before you were born.** Studies have shown that stress-induced high levels of cortisol in a pregnant woman can affect the development of the fetus. If the mother's cortisol is high, her baby will also have high levels of this stress hormone. The elevated cortisol level in the fetus can alter the receptors for stress-related substances in the brain, making those receptors more sensitive to stress for the child's entire life. Many diseases that appear in midlife, like diabetes and high blood pressure, are more common in adults who experienced stress in the womb or in the early period after birth. Knowing how your stress can mold an unborn child should motivate you to learn how to de-stress before you even consider having a child. You may also want to help pregnant women you love—your friends, daughter, daughter-in-law, colleagues—to relax. Our global future depends on healthy mothers and women.

The way you are raised also has a major effect on how you respond to stress. As a child, you learned your coping skills from your parents: you saw how they behaved in stressful situations and subconsciously shaped your behavior according to what you observed. In some cases, however, children who watched parents deal with the world in a dysfunctional way do everything they can to avoid acting like their parents. Take the case of an explosively angry parent. A child might be so terrorized by her parent's violent temper that she avoids any conflict. This, too, can be detrimental if she can't stand up for herself or her point of view.

In addition, genetic predisposition plays a big role in determining your stress response. The Human Genome Project analyzed forty-five stress-related markers and several important genomic switches that turn on the stress response in our bodies. These scientists had expected to find significant individual differences among their subjects, but they had not anticipated the wide range of variation they found.

Dr. Barry Bittman, the principal investigator on one of the Human Genome Project's stress studies, speculated that each person in his study had a distinctive genomic fingerprint for stress response. Two statisticians tested his theory from several different mathematical perspectives and arrived at the same conclusions. Dr. Bittman and his colleagues coined the term *individualized genomic stress-induction signatures* to describe the unique physiological and psychological response to stress that each of us has. We prefer to call it a fingerprint.

At this time, we simply don't know how much of the stress response is determined genetically, but scientists agree that every person possesses a genetically determined personal chemistry that is responsible for his or her in-born temperament. Your genetic inheritance and your experience create your personality—the way you feel, think, and behave. In turn, your values, goals, and beliefs about yourself and the world contribute to how you manage potential adversity—and stress.

## THE EMOTIONS OF STRESS

According to psychologist Daniel Goleman, emotions are impulses to act, "instant plans for handling life." Emotions help you to deal with a threatening situation by short-cutting your intellect; your body acts to protect you more quickly than if you took the time to reflect on a situation. When you experience a stress emotion, you usually know immediately that you have to pay attention to a situation—even if you rationally choose not to act and even if you have time to try to approach the situation intellectually. Psychologist Richard Lazarus outlined six broad situations that create stress-inducing emotions:

- The situation has to be relevant to what you want. The more important a goal is to you, the more intense your emotion will be.
- The situation threatens your achieving what you want. Negative emotions will emerge when your goals are being frustrated.
- Something important to you is being threatened. If your self-esteem, the positive opinion of others, your ideals, moral values or beliefs, people you love, or objects you value are threatened, you will feel stress.
- You blame yourself or others for a bad situation. If you take on blame, you will experience guilt, shame, and anger at yourself. If you blame others, you will be angry.
- You feel that a bad situation is beyond your control or that you will not be able to cope. Feeling powerless or overwhelmed always leads to stress.
- You sense that things will not work out in your favor. Having expectations that the situation will turn out badly will obviously result in negative emotions.

> *Adapted from www.mindtools.com/stress/rt/EmotionalAnalysis .htm. Reproduced with permission. Copyright © Mind Tools Ltd, 1995–2008, All Rights Reserved.*

These situations produce emotions that can trigger a physical stress response, putting your body into overdrive. Feeling anger, anxiety, fear, guilt, shame, sadness, grief, envy, or jealousy can dramatically disrupt your body's balance, depending on the intensity of these emotions.

Hyperactive stress responders, who are always intense, are more prone to anger, anxiety, envy, jealousy, and optimism, while hypoactive stress responders are more likely to turn their feelings inward and are more prone to sadness, fear, guilt, shame, hopelessness, and pessimism.

Another thing to remember that might help you when you are in a stressful situation is that when you are chronically stressed, your thinking can become distorted and you can assess stressors to be more of a threat than they are. **You can actually create stress simply by anticipating a stressful situation.**

Let's say you overslept on the morning of a departmental meeting. There is no way you can make it on time. You have to decide if you should call in sick, whether you should rush and draw attention to yourself by walking into the conference room in the middle of the meeting, or if you should slip into work and skip the meeting. Your decision and stress level might be based on whether you are essential to the meeting, if you feel secure in your job, whether the climate in your office is informal or corporate, or your relationship with your boss and colleagues.

If your primary appraisal—deciding whether you are in a situation that will harm or help you—finds the circumstance stressful, you automatically shift to secondary appraisal, in which you determine if anything can be done to alter the situation; in this process, you consider whether a coping strategy will be effective. You then must decide whether you have the resources to produce the outcome you want; those resources include social and problem-solving skills, energy, health, education, and money, to name just a few.

To return to the meeting dilemma, you might feel confident about your position in the company and know your boss will understand and accept your apology when you show up. You could call your boss's assistant and ask him to give her a message that you have been delayed and will be there as soon as possible. If the office is formal and you don't get along well with your boss, you might want to avoid drawing attention to your being late by going to work, skipping the meeting, and apologizing later.

If your assessment is that your coping mechanisms are stronger than the threat, you are mobilized to eliminate or resolve the challenge. But if the risk is higher than you judge your coping skills to be, you can reduce the degree of the threat by escape or avoidance or you can prepare to deal with the situation by freezing momentarily. You might just throw in the towel and call in sick.

### A Challenge Becomes Stress When . . .

- The demands of a situation exceed your ability to cope with it.
- Your appraisal of the situation is inaccurate either because you overestimate what the situation demands or you underestimate your ability to cope.
- You exaggerate the consequences of not being able to cope with a situation.
- Expectations, beliefs, or fears keep you from using your coping skills.
- You lack an adequate support system.
- Inhibitions and fears keep you from using your support system.

In order to reduce stress, you have to understand what is causing the negative emotions that color your view. To do so, you need to step back from what you are experiencing to examine rationally what you are feeling. Of course, it is not always easy to separate your mind from a strong emotion. In this chapter, we give you the tools to analyze what you are feeling and to quiet these draining, stress-inducing emotions. We want to show you how to recognize your feelings and break down your habits of thinking into smaller parts that will let you get control over your stress reaction.

## OPTIMISM V. PESSIMISM

The way you interpret events—the root of your expectations—is known as your "explanatory style." You judge the events in your life as good or bad, positive or negative. Optimists and pessimists differ in the way they respond to adversity. Are you one or the other, or a mix of both? Optimists are upbeat and confident that they can cope with most challenges; pessimists look on the dark side and always envision the worst-case scenario. A realistic sense of optimism can be energizing, but excessive optimism can deny reality and become counterproductive or self-sabotaging. A touch of pessimism can act as a good reality check, but the negative focus of extreme pessimism can be depressing. Before taking on a risky trip or dangerous project, you could benefit from using a pessimistic assessment with an optimistic attitude. Avoiding extremes is always preferable.

People with a pessimistic worldview tend to believe that their problems are pervasive and long-lasting, that those problems will undermine everything they do; they tend to blame themselves for their problems. In the same situations, optimists regard a problem as a temporary setback that is specific to that one situation, and not their fault. Given this dynamic, you can see how optimistic and pessimistic attitudes can become self-fulfilling prophecies. If you feel defeated from the start, you are not likely to take constructive action; your negative expectations will become your reality. If you consider a setback temporary, you will be more disposed to do something about it; because you act, you cause the situation to be temporary. Take a moment to reflect in your Stress Journal on your predominant attitude and whether optimism or pessimism prevails in all situations or whether you are optimistic at, say, work, but pessimistic with your family.

The impact that an optimistic or pessimistic outlook can have on your lifestyle is profound. Several large-scale, long-term, controlled experiments have found that optimists are more successful than pessimists—optimistic salespeople make more money; optimistic students get better grades; optimistic athletes win more events. Two studies of college students were conducted at the typically frenzied end of a semester, and both found that optimists reported fewer physical symptoms like headaches and colds than pessimists; if a person's expectations are negative, bad health often follows. Many studies have found that people who routinely respond to the stresses of life with depression, anxiety, hostility, and other displays of negative thinking are significantly less healthy. A meta-analysis of 101 studies confirmed that chronic anxiety, pessimism, cynicism, suspiciousness, and hostility are toxic. People who experienced any of these emotions over a long period had double the risk of diseases like arthritis, asthma, headaches, peptic ulcers, and heart disease.

### From the Bench

**PESSIMISM AND YOUR HEALTH**

Harvard clinical psychologist Dr. Martin Seligman, author of *Learned Optimism*, conducted a now-famous longitudinal study of Harvard University graduates. He and his colleagues found that those men who had a pessimistic explanatory style at the age of twenty-five had significantly worse health or were more likely to have died when they were assessed twenty to thirty-five years later.

One of the psychological side effects of chronic stress is increased negativity, hopelessness, and pessimism. The more stress you are under, the more negatively you think, which of course creates more stress. Excessive pessimism stresses your body internally, because a pessimist's stress response is triggered more often and stays switched on longer than an optimist's. Hopelessness decreases the resistance to stress and increases mental and physical vulnerability. When people think they are powerless to influence events, they do not act to improve their situations, because they are certain of failure before they have begun. **Negative thinking undermines your confidence and your quality of life.**

Please take a minute to check in with yourself in your Stress Journal and note situations in which you have had negative thoughts. Write down the kinds of situations, thoughts, and what happened.

## STRESSFUL CORE BELIEFS AND "CROOKED THINKING"

You use a set of beliefs to interpret everything that happens to you. These core beliefs developed as you interacted with the world and learned from your parents, friends, school, culture, religion, media, and the arts. Your beliefs define you even though their influence is often unconscious and even if your beliefs do not necessarily reflect reality. **Beliefs are opinions, not facts.** It is essential that you examine your thoughts and beliefs to see if they are based on reality. Stress-inducing beliefs almost always include the words *ought, should,* or *must.* Psychologist Albert Ellis referred to this sort of thinking as "should-izing": *My house should be immaculate. He should be nicer to me. I ought to make a higher salary. I must finish everything I have to do.* Should-izing creates an enormous amount of stress and guilt. In 1975, Albert Ellis created a list of the most common misconceptions and core beliefs that can provoke a stress response, and that list has been expanded over the years. These beliefs and irrational ideas can limit your experience of life and will most likely produce frustration and negativity.

Cognitive distortions in your thought processes, which Albert Ellis called "crooked thinking," contribute to your perception of a stressful situation. Simply recognizing these irrational modes of thought as automatic distortions of reality in your mind-set helps you to reduce stress. You might respond to a situation with high levels of stress, because you make faulty assumptions and your responses are inappropriately governed by false interpretations.

What follows is a list of the most common core beliefs and forms of "crooked thinking" that can lead to a physical stress response. As you read through this list, be aware of your inner voice. Identify the beliefs and thought patterns that shape your reaction to people and the world around you—in short, your reality. Please record your limiting core beliefs and cognitive distortions in your Stress Journal. We'll return to them later as we teach you techniques to control your stress response.

**Demand for Approval:** You measure your worth by how well other people treat you. You need the constant love and approval of people who are important to you.

**High Self-expectations:** You are achievement-oriented and must be successful in everything you do. You demand a lot from yourself and have a hard time forgiving yourself if anything you do is less than excellent.

**Emotional Control:** You are overly sensitive to the opinions and judgments of others. You allow what you imagine other people think of you to dictate your decisions, even if it means not doing or going after what you want.

**Dependency:** You believe you are unable to cope with life by yourself and must depend on someone smarter or stronger than yourself. You feel powerless to solve your own problems and rely on others to take care of them.

**Helplessness:** You think there is nothing you can do to solve your problems, whether they are of your own making or were caused by an external situation, and haven't accepted that the capacity to change is in all of us.

**Fairness Fallacy:** You believe that the world and everyone in it must be fair and just.

**Avoidance:** Rather than confront difficulties and responsibilities directly, you avoid facing them.

**Discomfort Anxiety:** You don't believe in rocking the boat or pushing yourself, because you are not willing to risk pain and anxiety. This limiting attitude can keep you from doing things outside your comfort zone from which you could benefit.

**Perfectionism:** You believe that there is a perfect solution to every problem. You think everything should work better or go more smoothly. You judge others with very rigid standards.

**Fear of Losing Control:** When you are under stress, you fear that you're "losing it" or that you are going crazy. You fear you might have a breakdown and cannot imagine how to pull the pieces back together.

**All-or-nothing Thinking:** No middle ground exists with this sort of thinking. Situations are good or bad, opinions are right or wrong, your efforts result in success or utter failure.

**Catastrophizing:** The assumption that the worst will always happen fills you with dread and makes you doubt your ability to cope.

**Keeping the Negatives:** You perceive only the negatives in a situation and ignore the positives. You obsess about bad comments and perceived slights.

**Magnifying or Minimizing:** You tend to lose your sense of proportion. You inflate the importance of minor things. You blow up your weaknesses and minimize your strengths.

**Personalization:** When something goes wrong, you feel you are totally responsible.

**Jumping to Conclusions:** This type of crooked thinking takes two forms:
   **Fortune-telling:** You are certain how things will turn out even if you have no facts to support your prediction.
   **Mind reading:** You think you know what other people are thinking, and it's usually negative about you.

**Emotional Reasoning:** Your feelings, rather than facts, dominate your interpretations.

**Hindsight:** Though it's a normal part of the learning process to look back to learn from your mistakes, you are preoccupied with mistakes you made in the past, which limits your thinking and behavior in the present and creates stress in new situations.

**What-ifs:** Focusing on the worst possible outcome can prevent you from assessing a situation accurately and determining a practical course of action. Considering possibilities is important but, if taken to an extreme, can muddy your thinking and prevent you from taking appropriate action.

**Egocentric Thinking:** You feel the need to persuade others to believe what you believe. You want to influence what others think.

**Control Error:** You either feel responsible for everything or you feel helpless to change anything.

**Heaven's Reward Thinking:** You put others' needs first, because you believe that you will gain your reward in the future.

**Unrealistic Comparisons:** You compare yourself to others and automatically judge them to be smarter, more successful, happier than you are.

All these inaccurate attitudes and assumptions set you up for chronic frustration. They are guaranteed to take the joy out of life. Do you recognize some of your beliefs and ways of interacting with the world? Take a step back and think about what that little voice in your head is actually doing for you. Is your inner voice articulating a false belief? How automatically does that false belief pop into your mind? Think about how it makes you feel and about whether it serves you well when it comes to decision time. If you can understand that your belief causes you to overreact and that it is creating stress, you can prevent your body from shifting into stress mode.

Your first step to reducing your stress is this exercise in recognizing how your assumptions and reactions contribute to or perhaps even cause your stress. When an event triggers these thought patterns and stress-inducing core beliefs, you will feel negative emotions—anger, anxiety, fright, guilt, shame, sadness—all of which can lead to a greater sense of stress. But once you begin to become aware of your automatic responses, you can also learn to stop them.

## CHALLENGING CORE BELIEFS AND DISTORTED THOUGHTS

Irrational beliefs fall into four general categories:

- Absolutes—musts and shoulds
- Awfulizing—exaggerated negativity
- Can't stand its
- Being highly critical of yourself or others

If you recognize some of these beliefs in your thought patterns, make an effort to stop yourself when you hear that little voice in your head. Is your inner voice articulating a true belief? Take a moment to notice how automatic that response is. Think about how the belief is making you feel. Finally, judge whether your belief is realistic or overly rigid

**Checklist for Challenging Core Beliefs**

What is the real-world evidence?

Am I making a mistake about what causes what?

Am I confusing a thought with a fact?

Am I using absolutes—musts and shoulds?

Am I taking examples out of context?

Am I being honest with myself?

What is the source of the information?

Am I assessing the chance of something happening too high or too low?

Am I assuming that every situation is the same?

Am I focusing on irrelevant factors?

Am I overlooking my strengths?

Am I concentrating on my weaknesses?

What do I want?

What can I do to solve the problem?

How would I look at this from someone else's point of view?

Am I asking myself questions that have no answers, such as, "Why did this happen to me?"

What are the advantages of thinking this way?

What are the disadvantages of thinking this way?

What difference will this make in a week, a year, ten years?

*Adapted from* Getting Undepressed, *by Gary Emery, PhD*

in a particular situation. If you can understand and accept how your belief is causing you to overreact to an event, creating stress, you are in a position to defuse your stress response. If you can challenge a core belief, you will be able to change that belief consciously so that you can respond productively to life's upsets.

## THE ABC MODEL

Besides his list of "crooked thinking," Dr. Albert Ellis also created Rational Emotive Behavioral Therapy, which uses your rational understanding of your emotions to help you change your behavior. It's a long name for an elegantly simple way to help identify the role that beliefs, thoughts, and emotions play in triggering a stress response. He calls this process the A+B=C equation.

> **Activating Event + Beliefs = Consequences**

With a little practice, you will be able to break down your reaction to a situation from a rational point of view. To start, we suggest that you keep a log in your Stress Journal of what sets you off, what buttons that event is pushing, and what emotions you feel. This record will give you insight into how your thoughts and beliefs are responsible for the negative emotions that trigger your stress response.

| **A** | **B** | **C** |
|---|---|---|
| **Activating Event or Trigger** | **Beliefs** | **Consequences** |
| *Write down an event or situation that is triggering or has triggered stress.* | *Record the thoughts that are going through or have gone through your head.* | *List the feelings you are experiencing or have experienced.* |
| Getting lost on the way to an interview | Everything always goes wrong.<br><br>I always get lost. I have a terrible sense of direction.<br><br>The directions they gave me are just not clear enough.<br><br>I'll never get that job if I'm late. | Anxiety<br>Frustration<br>Worry<br>Anger |
| Overcooking a dish for a dinner party | I'm a lousy cook and never should have tried that hard recipe.<br><br>If my husband had only helped with something, for a change, this wouldn't have happened.<br><br>I can't cope—what do I say to our guests?<br><br>Our guests will have an awful time and will think I'm a terrible hostess. | Frustration<br>Guilt<br>Anger<br>Anxiety<br>Embarrassment<br>Shame |
| Your son is late coming home from a date. | What if he had a horrible car wreck?<br><br>He is so inconsiderate not to call to let me know where he is.<br><br>Maybe he's just ignoring his curfew. I'm just not strict enough.<br><br>What if he's been drinking at the party and is too out of it to call to say he can't drive? He wouldn't get into the car in that condition, would he? | Fear<br>Anxiety<br>Anger<br>Worry |

| You are not asked to attend a meeting at the office. | Being left out is a disaster. | Anxiety |
| --- | --- | --- |
| | I'm not important enough. | Shame |
| | My supervisor must hate me. | Fear |
| | I just don't measure up. | Worry |
| | This must mean I'm on my way out. | |

# IT'S YOUR CHOICE

As you break down your reaction to a situation with your "emotional ABCs," you're basically reorganizing the way you think—and this will help you to moderate your stress response. Next, we will take you step-by-step through a method that will help you to develop a flexible, accurate style of thinking—called "cognitive restructuring"—that will help you reduce your stress further.

Since your stress responses are generated by your interpretations of events, cognitive restructuring eases stress by showing you how to evaluate whether your interpretations are valid or not. You reframe stress-inducing emotional reactions, determine whether your reaction is warranted, and then break the habit of thinking negatively. You replace stress-making thought patterns with a balanced point of view, which is also healthier and more positive. You choose to apply rationality to emotions that are triggered by stressful situations. It might sound as if we are asking you to accomplish a major shift in your thinking, but with a bit of practice it is surprisingly easy to alter your response patterns to incorporate this stress-reducing method. Cognitive restructuring helps you to see a situation accurately.

### Cognitive Restructuring
  1. Become aware of harmful core beliefs and negative thought patterns.

2. Challenge those stress-inducing mind-sets.
3. Replace them with healthy, affirming, balanced thoughts and beliefs.

## COGNITIVE REAPPRAISAL WORKS

Researchers at Stanford University studied MRI brain images of two groups of people as they watched a terrifying movie in order to compare two methods of regulating emotions—cognitive reappraisal or suppression of emotion. Cognitive reappraisal reduced the intensity of negative emotions, while suppression of emotions actually increased the intensity of brain response. In other words, the study reveals that if you do not deal with your negative emotions, the intensity of those emotions only increases. Learning to reframe your thinking will help you to regulate your negative emotions and reduce your stress.

In a separate, Swiss study, men and women who underwent cognitive behavioral stress-management training for four months showed significantly reduced cortisol stress responses—again, reframing reduced stress.

## ABCDE COGNITIVE RESTRUCTURING

Adding two more steps to the process of examining your reactions to events will help you determine whether your thoughts are accurate and whether there is anything you can do to change the triggering event or your reaction to it. At this stage of the process, you may learn that your core beliefs and thinking patterns are not necessarily reliable and can cause you to interpret a situation incorrectly or deal with it ineffectively. Once you understand why you are experiencing a certain emotion, you will have to D, dispute your automatic negative thoughts by considering a positive alternative. Then you have to consider E, effective new approaches to cope with the situation. Doing this will help you to restructure your thinking and develop better coping strategies. This process is designed to make you aware of dysfunctional beliefs and mind-sets and help you to correct them. Cognitive therapy is action-oriented to solve problems, which in turn will relieve your stress. You can work on restructuring during a scheduled journaling time. You will eventually see what alternatives and solutions work best for you to resolve your problems and to reduce your stress.

Let's apply these additional steps to the sample ABC log.

| A<br><br>Activating Event or Trigger<br><br>*Write down an event or situation that is triggering or has triggered stress.* | B<br><br>Beliefs<br><br>*Record the thoughts that are going through or have gone through your head.* | C<br><br>Consequences<br><br>*List the feelings you are experiencing or have experienced.* | D<br><br>Dispute<br><br>*Positive alternative to automatic negative thought* | E<br><br>Energize with effective new approaches |
|---|---|---|---|---|
| Getting lost on the way to an interview. | Everything always goes wrong.<br><br>I always get lost.<br><br>I have a terrible sense of direction.<br><br>The directions they gave me are just not clear enough.<br><br>I'll never get that job if I'm late. | Anxious<br><br>Frustrated<br><br>Worried<br><br>Angry | Things do not always go wrong.<br><br>Everyone gets lost now and then, even the interviewer.<br><br>Even if being late is a strike against me, I'll have to be more impressive.<br><br>The company gives these directions to many people. They are likely to be correct. I should pull over to read them carefully.<br><br>Maybe the interviewer is running late. | If I am running late, I will pull over and call to let the person I am meeting know that I have been delayed.<br><br>When I have to go to an important appointment, I will do a dry run first to make sure I know how to get there.<br><br>I'll save for a GPS system. Having one would wipe out a major source of stress in my life. |

(*continued on next page*)

| A | B | C | D | E |
|---|---|---|---|---|
| **Activating Event or Trigger** | **Beliefs** | **Consequences** | **Dispute** | **Energize with effective new approaches** |
| *Write down an event or situation that is triggering or has triggered stress.* | *Record the thoughts that are going through or have gone through your head.* | *List the feelings you are experiencing or have experienced.* | *Positive alternative to automatic negative thought* | |
| Overcooking a complicated dish for a dinner party. | I'm a lousy cook. I never should have tried that hard recipe. If my husband had only helped with something, this wouldn't have happened. I can't cope—what do I say to our guests? Our guests will have an awful time and will think I'm a terrible hostess. | Frustrated Guilty Angry Anxious Embarrassed Ashamed | You have turned out some great meals. Are you being a perfectionist? Is the dish servable? If you have no help, you have to manage your time better. Everyone has had a disaster in the kitchen. Your guests will understand, and most people won't notice it's off. This is only one part of the meal. The rest will be delicious. | Try a new recipe before using it for a dinner party. Either ask for help in advance or manage your time better. Be flexible enough to throw something simple together if a dish is ruined. Keep your sense of humor—your guests are there for more than the food. |
| Your son is late coming home from a date. | What if he had a horrible car wreck? He must be hurt since he hasn't called. Maybe he's just ignoring his curfew. I'm just not strict enough. | Frightened Anxious Angry Worried | He has been late before without having had an accident. The police would have called had he been hurt. All kids come home late now and then. | Establish rules for letting you know when he will be late, with consequences if breaks curfew without calling. |

| | | | | |
|---|---|---|---|---|
| | Or he could have been drinking at the party and is too out of it to call to say he can't drive.<br>He wouldn't get into the car in that condition, would he? | | Maybe he is just having a good time.<br>It is better if he stays at the party to sober up if he has been drinking. | Come to an understanding that he should stay where he is rather than drive while under the influence, but to let you know he will be late. |
| You are not asked to attend a meeting at the office. | Being left out is a disaster.<br>I'm not important enough.<br>My supervisor must hate me.<br>I just don't measure up.<br>This must mean I'm on my way out. | Anxious<br>Ashamed<br>Frightened<br>Worried | Does everyone always attend all meetings?<br>There are so many meetings that missing one is not a crisis.<br>Have others at your level been asked to attend?<br>The meeting might have nothing to do with your area of expertise.<br>Not being included does not necessarily reflect your supervisor's opinion of you. | View not having to attend the meeting as found time to catch up.<br>Ask your supervisor if you can attend the meeting or offer to take notes.<br>Ask your supervisor if it is appropriate for you to have a look at the meeting notes. |

The process is very straightforward. If you find that you have been stressed out by a situation, take a time-out to consider what is bothering you. Ask yourself these questions:

### ABCDE Questions

| | |
|---|---|
| How do I feel? | Emotion |
| What am I thinking? | Self-talk |
| What core beliefs are influencing my perception of what happened? | Core beliefs |

| | |
|---|---|
| Are any cognitive distortions contributing to my stressful response? | Crooked thinking |
| Do my assumptions accurately reflect what happened? | Challenge |
| Do the facts support my interpretation? | Challenge |
| Is there a more positive way to interpret the event? | Reappraisal |
| If I'm right, what is the worst that can happen? | Reappraisal |
| Am I underestimating my ability to handle the consequences of the event? | Reappraisal |
| What can I do to improve the situation? | Coping |

When you use cognitive restructuring, you will gain insight into how your thinking sets off and exacerbates your stress response. Rational understanding is the first step. It takes persistence and practice, but this method will allow you to replace negative, self-sabotaging thoughts with affirming, healthy ones that will boost your sense of well-being. If you find yourself struggling to maintain these practices, you might want to talk through a problem with a close friend using these techniques; having another point of view can give you important insights and take you out of yourself and your point of view. A support network of sympathetic friends and family will make the process easier. Working through your problems with a friend will also satisfy the tend-and-befriend response. We will discuss this primal stress reaction, which is particulary important for women, in the next chapter. You can reciprocate and help a friend restructure her reactions.

The use of cognitive restructuring can keep your exchanges from becoming emotional rants that accomplish little. If your stress and problems seem insurmountable, consider working with a therapist trained in cognitive therapy. A professional therapist can help anyone make the process of change more efficient and longer lasting.

## STRESS-HARDINESS

Awareness of your negative beliefs alone is a good start to reducing your stress, but it is often not enough. These beliefs and thought patterns are deeply ingrained, and changing them usually takes effort; unless you are one of the few women we have seen who seem resistant to stress and who are able to adjust to change with ease, responding to stressful situations in an adaptive, effective way. Dr. Suzanne Kobasa, a psychologist, identifies this style of coping as "hardiness." Stress-hardiness is not the avoidance of stress so much as it is a positive response to stressful situations and a self-efficacy that minimizes negative effects. The good news is that you can learn to become stress-hardy at any stage of life. Gaining this outlook and adaptability can change the relationship between stress and illness.

## THE ELEMENTS OF RESILIENCE AND STRESS-HARDINESS

Studying business executives over a period of eight years, Dr. Kobasa found three personality traits in those who remained the healthiest as their company underwent a major restructuring. She found that these traits protected some of the executives and managers from the physiological effects of stress. Dr. Kobasa measured emotional response to stressful situations, including depressed mood, anxiety, displeasure, and anger. She also studied cognitive and behavioral responses—loss of confidence, distrust, despair, worry, unrealistic wishes, inactivity, withdrawal, and impatience. She discovered three components of hardiness. As you would expect, people who possess these traits have lower negative responses to stress. To give you a sense of what it takes to deal with stress in a healthy way, here are the three traits of stress-hardiness.

## COMMITMENT

Commitment means having a sense of purpose for why you are doing what you are doing. It means being involved in family, work, and having a social network. It may also mean that you have a religious faith and are rooted in strong personal values. This sort of involvement supports you in solving your problems without letting stress disrupt your goals. Commitment also means dedication to a task and the belief that it is achievable.

## CONTROL

The need for too much control can be a source of stress. There are two types of control, internal and external. People who have an internal locus of control know that they cannot influence all the external events that occur in their lives, but they feel that they have a choice in how they react to those stressors. Those who have an external locus of control believe that they have little control over what happens to them, and that fate or destiny dictates their circumstances.

When you have a healthy perspective on control, you focus your efforts on events you can influence and do not worry about things beyond your control. You believe you can actively chart the course of your life by solving problems and making decisions. Even if it does not work out as planned, at least you have not passively accepted something that makes you unhappy. The knowledge that you cannot control every detail of your life and the awareness of what you can control are significant stress reducers. The Serenity Prayer, adapted by Alcoholics Anonymous and other twelve-step movements, eloquently captures the ideal frame of mind.

**The Serenity Prayer**

God grant us the serenity to accept the things we cannot change, courage to change the things we can, and wisdom to know the difference.

## CHALLENGE

Challenge is really a mind-set about change. Stress-hardy people are not frightened by change because they regard it as an opportunity to learn and to grow. They view change as a challenge that they want to confront and control rather than a stress to avoid. They are willing

**Portrait of a Stress-hardy Woman**

- A sense of meaning, direction, and purpose animates her life.

- Her values guide her rather than her emotions. She views emotions as a source of energy and motivation but understands that emotions are not reliable guides.

- She knows how to motivate herself to take action and concentrates on what she wants, not on what she doesn't want.

- She has a strong social network and relies reasonably on the support of others.

- When things go wrong, she doesn't judge herself or others harshly.

- She has a sense of humor and is reasonably optimistic. She doesn't take herself too seriously.

- She evaluates her ways of thinking and behaving and makes changes if they are not working.

- She views adversity as a challenge rather than a threat. She knows she will grow and learn from whatever happens.

- She looks for solutions that work for everyone.

- She knows how to mourn life's inevitable losses.

- She is able to let go of things she has no control over.

- She is grateful for the good things in her life.

*Adapted from a compilation by Jean Browman, stresstopower.com, cheerfulmonk.com* to work through difficult circumstances and even look forward to the chance to think creatively.

In the end, you cannot avoid stress, but you can learn to respond to it in the most positive manner and minimize its negative effects.

With your understanding of how your perceptions influence your stress reaction, you can now draw from your reservoir of resilience. The next step is to take a close look at what actually goes on in your body in response to stress. Chapter 3, "The Anatomy of Stress," will give you an understanding of the ancient survival mechanism that is activated in your body when you sense a threat and how chronic stress throws you out of balance.

# CHAPTER THREE

# THE ANATOMY OF STRESS

A s women, we often believe that life will be smooth sailing when we finish that last chore, pay off our mortgage, get that promotion, have enough money in the bank, see our children solve their problems and thrive, or lose that last ten pounds. But those are unrealistic expectations. Peace and contentment are transient states. Life is going to throw new challenges at you almost every day. Meeting these challenges and coping with them is what living is all about.

The same dynamic—this process of adaptation—goes on in a very complex way within your brain and body to allow you to evaluate and respond to the countless external and internal challenges you encounter every day. Your brain directs the adjustments—both subtle and dramatic—that are necessary for you to maintain homeostasis, a steady internal state. Since your circumstances change moment by moment, your various body systems cooperate to maintain balance and to operate within an acceptable range of parameters. The adaptive responses that your body makes to keep your internal environment stable occur at the systemic and cellular levels. Your body temperature, the rate at which your heart beats, and the amount of oxygen in your blood are all regulated by an integrated network of systems that work in continuous dynamic balance, making minute adjustments and countless corrections to stay the course.

In this chapter, we give you an overview of how these intricate systems function and communicate to protect you from harm and to ensure your survival. As doctors, we have come to view our female bodies and biology as masterpieces, living works of art. The dynamic balance we are able to maintain surpasses even the most vivid moment captured on a canvas, which is always static. Each of us is the curator

---

## From the Bench

### A BRIEF HISTORY OF STRESS

Stress has been a subject of speculation and study since the time of the ancient Greeks. We have condensed the evolving scientific thinking on stress to show you how science builds on itself over time. We are on the brink of a deeper understanding of the intricate systems of checks and balances that operate in you to maintain homeostasis.

#### ANCIENT GREEKS

**Empedocles** made the first written reference to *homeostasis*, a steady state of harmony, balance, and equilibrium in the body.

**Hippocrates** considered *health a harmonious balance and disease a disharmony* caused by disturbing forces of nature.

**Epicurus** recognized the *psychological causes of stress* and wrote that coping with emotional stress could improve the quality of life.

#### EARLY NINETEENTH CENTURY

**Claude Bernard** and the *milieu interieur*—discovered that the more complex an organism, the more complex adaptive mechanisms have to become to keep the *milieu interieur*, or inner environment, constant.

#### 1914

**Walter Cannon** conducted experiments that identified the *fight-or-flight response* and the physiology behind it. He found that *physical and emotional challenges triggered the same response*. He discovered that there was a critical level of stress, based on the magnitude and duration of the stressor, that would cause the homeostatic mechanisms to fail.

1924

**W. R. Hess** (Nobel laureate) used the terms *ergotropic* and *trophotropic* to distinguish between the roles of the *sympathetic* and *parasympathetic* systems of the autonomic nervous system as they interact with psychological processes and physical responses to adapt to the demands of the environment.

1936

**Hans Seyle** identified a three-stage reaction to stress that he called the *general adaptation syndrome*. He believed that the general adaptation syndrome involved primarily the nervous and endocrine (or hormone) systems. The three stages of the stress response he delineated are: alarm, when the threat is identified; resistance, when the body attempts to cope with the stress; and exhaustion, when the body's resources are depleted, functioning is no longer normal, and long-term damage can occur.

CONTEMPORARY

**James Henry, MD,** explored and introduced the significance of perception and anxiety in activating the stress response.

**Peter S. Sterling and Joseph Eyer,** of the University of Pennsylvania, were pioneers in combining the disciplines of social science and medicine. They created the term *allostasis*. *Allostasis* refers to the intricate and active processes by which an organism maintains stability, or homeostasis, through adjustment and adaptation to predictable and unpredictable events. It is a more dynamic concept of balance than homeostasis.

**Shelley E. Taylor,** a psychologist at the University of California at Los Angeles, identified the *tend-and-befriend response* and the role of *oxytocin* as a stress response and survival mechanism, perhaps more important than the fight-or-flight response for women.

**Bruce McEwen,** head of the Neuroendocrinology Laboratory at Rockefeller University in New York City, coined the term *allostatic load*. Allostatic load refers to the wear and tear the brain and body experience with chronic stress.

of a priceless masterpiece, responsible for both its care and its restoration. That awareness still fills us with awe. We want you to feel the same way.

Chronic stress pushes your body to overreact, depletes your resources, and disrupts the balance that exists among these interconnected systems that are meant to protect you. In the broadest terms, stress puts a lot of wear and tear on the body that can be damaging. Chronic stress can impair growth and development and lead to metabolic, immune, hormonal, and psychiatric disorders. Whether such conditions occur depends on your genetic vulnerability, the type of stress you have been exposed to, and the duration and timing of stressful events. We are all more vulnerable to stressors at certain critical periods in the womb, infancy, childhood, and adolescence. The neural pathways are still developing at those times and can become permanently altered by traumatic or repeated stress.

# ALLOSTASIS

*Allostasis* is a recently coined term that refers to your body's process of maintaining optimum stability and efficiency when dealing with predictable and unpredictable events in your life. Allostatic systems help you to adapt by adjusting themselves in response to your needs. Simply put, any living being must be able to evaluate, respond, and adjust to the demands of its environment. The more complex the organism and its environment, the more intricate and multifaceted the process of allostasis has to be.

The process of allostasis is at work in you all the time. It requires constant communication between your brain and your body. This dynamic cross talk can be finely tuned when subtle adjustments are appropriate or fully activated when necessary. Acute stress sets off an emergency alarm that disrupts allostatic balance.

A perfect example of allostasis at work during a predictable event occurs when you wake up in the morning. Going from sleep to awareness is a routine event you take for granted. It is not the simple process it appears to be. A number of highly orchestrated interactions between your brain and your body are set in motion when your inner clock determines that it is time to awaken. Increases in your blood pressure and heart rate allow you to stand up, and energy has been mobilized in anticipation of your awakening and moving around. At the same time as your brain has directed these changes, your brain is shifting from a dream state to alert perception of the world around you. This transition is achieved seamlessly as various systems collaborate and balance one another to establish this goal.

## THE FIGHT-OR-FLIGHT RESPONSE

Acute stress stimulates a powerful series of responses in your body designed to help you survive a threatening situation. This is allostasis in the extreme. The body's response to acute stress was identified by Walter Cannon in 1915 when he described how animals reacted to threats. Known as the "fight-or-flight response," this survival mechanism provides a powerful, almost instantaneous reaction to an emergency that gets maximum energy to the parts of the body that need it most. Automatic and primitive, the response is hardwired into your brain to provide immediate protection from bodily harm. When your brain perceives danger, a sequence of dramatic changes occurs in your allostatic pathways that prepare your body for action:

- Pupils dilate to improve vision, awareness intensifies.
- Heart rate increases.
- Blood vessels in the skin constrict to avoid blood loss in case of injury, which is responsible for the feeling that your hair is standing on end.
- Increased blood supply goes to peripheral muscles, while the systems that are not essential for immediate survival temporarily shut down. For example, production of saliva is reduced, one of the reasons why you experience dry mouth when you get up to speak in front of an audience.

- Breathing speeds up to increase oxygen in the blood.
- Fat from fat cells and glucose from the liver are metabolized for instant energy.
- Sweat glands open, providing a coolant for an overworked system.
- Endorphins—natural painkillers—are released.

The fight-or-flight response creates a state of arousal and vigilance that provides extra energy to accomplish extraordinary things, but it can also be damaging and accelerate disease. With chronic stress, the very system designed to help you survive a threat can itself become the threat, if not properly controlled. Stress researchers today interpret certain forms of coping as fight-or-flight—including social withdrawal and alcohol and drug abuse. The subjective experience of fight-or-flight is arousal, fear, and anxiety.

In order for you to understand our types and the goals of our Stress Detox Programs, we have to take a closer look at what happens in your body in response to a perceived state of emergency.

## LIFE AS A FIRE DRILL

Allostasis is a state of optimum balance and function. With acute stress, emotional or physical, the focus of your brain and body changes dramatically. Mental alertness and memory increase, and the immune system is activated to defend against trauma or infection. Muscles tense in preparation for action, and the heart beats faster. All this requires a large energy expenditure and is debilitating if maintained for too long a period of time or if activated too frequently. This complicated and elaborate process is carefully monitored and controlled by the brain. At the same time as the stress response is initiated, many other pathways are activated in the brain that allow for repair and restoration after the stressful situation has resolved. If these balancing pathways are weak or ineffective, proper restoration cannot occur.

The fight-or-flight response is set off by the most primitive part of your brain, where responses are automatic. It is an appropriate response for a situation of immediate and grave danger. Fight-or-flight developed to deal with short periods of physical stress. These dramatic physical changes are not necessary to respond effectively to modern stressors, which are often emotional and psychological in nature and do not require these large bursts of energy to resolve. With modern stress, we activate emergency reactions far more often than necessary. We are experiencing change at an unprecedented pace, and the modern lifestyle has pushed us beyond our biological limits to cope. Fight-or-flight is not an ideal system for dealing with work stress or unpaid

## From the Bench

### EVEN OUR EMOTIONS ARE SOCIALLY DETERMINED

Walter Cannon and Phillip Bard, of Harvard, developed a theory of emotion that was refined by Stanley Schecter and Jerome Singer in the 1960s. The Cannon-Bard theory holds that emotions are formed when the brain assesses general states of arousal and assigns an emotion to the aroused physical state.

Schecter and Singer built on this theory by adding a social element to the creation of emotions. They believed that the brain and the social environment actually interact to form an emotion. The researchers designed a study to support their hypothesis: they injected the participants in the study with epinephrine to create an aroused state similar to what your body experiences with an activated fight-or-flight response. The participants were then sent to another room to wait with another person who appeared to be involved in the experiment as well. In fact, the other person was a research assistant who was instructed to act happy or angry. The real subjects reported feeling angry or happy during the experiment depending on the atmosphere created by the assistant with whom they spent time. Schecter and Singer concluded that when the brain receives the message that the body is aroused, it examines and judges the environment to choose an appropriate emotion. The reverse process is also true: an emotion can quickly move your body to a highly aroused state.

bills, but you might routinely activate this response, and it takes a serious toll on your physical and emotional health.

Fortunately, our brains are designed to control our primitive responses. This control originates in a part of the brain called the neocortex. It is the neocortex that makes us uniquely human. This region is particularly important in the "social" brains of humans. Human society requires a brain that is perceptive, adaptable, and able to make strategic decisions quickly. The neocortex is responsible for high-order thinking skills like reason, language, advanced planning, processing sensory information, and complex social interactions. In the response to stress, this part of your brain controls emotional and primitive responses like rage and anger. **Cognition trumps emotion in the human brain, allowing us to choose how we live and how we respond to stress.**

This is an example of how our brains operate on an interactive social level. Just as the perception of stress is a transaction between you and a stressor in your environment, as we described in chapter 2, our brains need a social context in order to appraise and make judgments. Our fundamentally social nature shapes our expectations and provides a backdrop for our evaluations.

## THE SOCIAL BRAIN

The relatively new field of social neuroscience is explaining how your social brain works. Your brain does not derive meaning simply by observing the outside world and arbitrarily assessing it by reflection or analysis. Scientists now believe that the human brain must exist in a world with shared social expectations, beliefs, and norms. We are not designed to exist in isolation.

One area of study that is receiving a good deal of attention is the role of mirror neurons in the brain. Mirror neurons play a significant role in allowing you to understand and to empathize with others. Your brain essentially reenacts in a muscle-specific way, without any actual muscle movement, what you have observed of someone you are watching. This "motor embodiment" allows us to feel what we would feel if we were actually making the same movement. The same is true when we perceive the emotions of others. Observing pain, happiness, or disgust activates regions in your brain involved in experiencing similar emotions, which enables you to understand and evaluate people more accurately. This mirroring produces a relationship between the observer and the observed. Mirror neurons create a reciprocal bond between social partners.

In social interaction, each person is both an observer and the one observed. Collaborating to achieve a goal together goes beyond simple actions. Goal sharing is an important property of the human mind and a key element of survival. The mirror-neuron system is at the core of our social nature and of how we perceive the world around us.

## THE STRESS RESPONSE

The brain is the central organ of stress. This is where stress originates. As the interpreter of your environment, it determines your immediate behavioral and physical response to a perceived threat or challenge. An intricate system of communication links your brain, autonomic nervous, hormone, and immune systems for internal defense and response. The brain sends messages to the autonomic nervous system and influences hormone production. The autonomic nervous system sends messages from the body to the brain. Important hormones integral to the stress response are produced within a part of the brain called the hypothalamus. Hormones then carry information to the brain, the autonomic nervous system, and the immune system. These are the pathways of integration that make the body and mind one in assessing and responding to our needs.

A two-part alarm system is set off in an acute response when allostasis is threatened: one activates the nervous system and the other is hormonal. The trigger for allostatic response begins in the hypothalamus with CRH (corticotropin-releasing hormone), which activates both systems. The alarm is sounded by a direct link from the brain to the adrenal glands, which produce a burst of epinephrine and norepinephrine for the fight-or-flight response. CRH also activates the HPA (hypothalamic-pituitary-adrenal) axis, which results in the release of the hormone cortisol from the adrenal glands. The hormone response lags slightly behind the epinephrine release of the neural response. In his pioneering work, Cannon identified these pathways as the sites of the physiological and psychological roots of stress. Although these two systems are intimately linked and aroused together with the stress response, they are functioning all the time to maintain allostasis and can function independently.

### The Messengers of the Stress Response

**CRH:** a hormone and neurotransmitter that stimulates the brain to release ACTH. An important communicator with the brain itself, CRH influences many levels of brain function.

**ACTH:** a hormone released in the brain that travels to the adrenal glands to stimulate production of cortisol.

**Cortisol:** the major stress hormone, produced in the adrenal glands, involved in the fight-or-flight response. It has significant influence on virtually all body functions, including brain activity, metabolism, and immune function.

**Norepinephrine (noradrenaline):** produced in the brain stem, this neurotransmitter activates the sympathetic nervous system, setting off the fight-or-flight response, and causes the adrenal glands to produce epinephrine. It affects arousal, attention, memory, improves mood, and growth of neural connections in the brain.

**Epinephrine (adrenaline):** produced in the adrenal glands and specialized sites in the brain, this neurotransmitter arouses the body and metabolizes glucose for energy supply.

**Oxytocin:** a brain hormone capable of buffering the fight-or-flight response. Oxytocin may be more significant in women's response to stress.

**Serotonin:** an important neurotransmitter that calms the stress response in the brain and influences appetite, mood, anger, fear, and aggression.

**Dopamine:** "the learning neurotransmitter" of the brain, is involved in many complex pathways, including reward, long-term memory, motivation, drug disorders, sleep, and motor systems.

**Endorphin:** a naturally occurring opiate-like neurotransmitter in the brain that decreases pain and enhances feelings of well-being. Endorphins may also play a significant role in the female response to stress.

## THE HPA AXIS

After the initial perception of a challenge or threat, the HPA (hypo-thalamic-pituitary-adrenal) axis comes into play. The HPA axis is the keystone of allostasis. With this process, your brain uses hormones as messengers to mobilize the system. The hypothalamus secretes CRH (corticotropin-releasing hormone), which travels in special blood vessels to the pituitary gland at the base of the brain. CRH signals the pituitary gland's release of ACTH (adrenocorticotropic hormone), which travels in the bloodstream to its primary target, the adrenal glands. The adrenal glands, located just above your kidneys, produce cortisol, the major stress hormone. Cortisol has effects on most of your allostatic pathways. Cortisol is essential for the normal function of your brain and body. It has a daily rhythm of ebb and flow, high in the morning and low at night. Too much or too little cortisol will affect how you look, how you sleep, your energy level, the quality of your emotions, and the function of your immune system.

## CORTISOL AND ABDOMINAL FAT

Cortisol is the culprit in the accumulation of fat around your middle. A key role of cortisol is to replenish energy supplies that are depleted by an acute stress response. Cortisol converts food into fat and stimulates appetite. An excess of cortisol also blocks insulin from stimulating the muscles to absorb glucose. Instead, the energy is stored as fat—especially around the middle. Abdominal fat is associated with insulin resistance, type 2 diabetes, heart disease, and inflammation. This is why reducing stress-induced cortisol levels is so important for your health.

## THE AUTONOMIC NERVOUS SYSTEM

The autonomic nervous system is the branch of the nervous system that controls involuntary responses. The autonomic nervous system links the brain stem, the most primitive part of the brain, by neural pathways that connect to target organs: the eyes, salivary glands, larynx, heart, lungs, stomach, intestines, and genitals. **The autonomic nervous system is divided into interacting and balancing systems, the sympathetic and parasympathetic nervous systems and the visceral afferent system.**

The sympathetic nervous system is activated by neurons in the primitive part of the brain called the brain stem. CRH, which jumpstarts the HPA axis during stress, also stimulates these neurons to produce norepinephrine. This neurotransmitter along with epinephrine mobilize the body for intense physical activity. Norepinephrine can also stimulate the release of CRH and an increased release of cortisol. These intricately linked systems are designed to interface and coordinate with each other. Imbalance in either system from chronic stress leads to disruption of allostasis.

Although we consider the autonomic nervous system a primitive part of the nervous system, it, too, is designed to function in a coordinated way. The sympathetic nervous system turns on the power and stimulates the body. A feedback network of nerves, known as the visceral afferent system, allows the brain to monitor the effects this stimulation has on critical parts of the body. A pounding heart, clenched stomach, and dry mouth are important signals to the brain. At the end of the stress, the brain activates the parasympathetic arm (PNS) of the autonomic nervous system. The PNS is designed to dampen the effects of the sympathetic nervous system and can turn off the emergency response. It restores the body to homeostasis and resets the priorities in the body to establish a balanced state. If a challenge persists without resolution, allostatic load or imbalance ensues.

The sympathetic and parasympathetic branches of the autonomic nervous system function in a fashion of dynamic opposition: arousal v. calm, energy mobilization v. energy storage, increased heart rate v. decreased heart rate. A balanced autonomic nervous system is essential for good physical and mental health. The only time the sympathetic and parasympathetic systems are active at the same time is during sexual arousal—which probably explains the power of sex.

## THE BRAIN UNDER STRESS

The interaction among parts of the brain and the communication of the brain with the body are accomplished by neurotransmitters, hormones, proteins, and immune messengers called cytokines, all of which carry information from one neuron to the next and from the nervous system to the hormone and immune systems. This communication is reciprocal. When the brain receives an arousal signal, it assesses the context of the arousal and determines the most appropriate emotion. One situation can elicit different results in emotional experience based on the social context. If fear is the perceived emotion, the sympathetic nervous system activates the primitive fight-or-flight response. Emotion and action are linked in this way.

What your brain chooses to set in motion in response to a perceived threat or challenge and what happens in the face of chronic stress are significantly influenced by what you have learned and remembered from previous experiences. The negative effects of stress on memory are complex. With chronic stress, it is not only harder to form new memories but more difficult to retrieve previously formed memories. Chronic stress can also interfere with neurogenesis, the formation of new neurons, and with neuroplasticity, the formation of new connections among neurons. Neuroplasticity is essential for the brain to create memories, to learn new tasks, and to make goal-directed decisions. Both of these processes are necessary for optimal brain function and to slow down the process of brain aging. This constant remodeling of our brains is what allows us to adapt to our ever-changing environment, which is the basis of allostasis. Flexibility, adaptability, and resilience are the result.

## TEND-AND-BEFRIEND

Many situations that arouse the stress response might not require a fight-or-flight reaction. Though you probably won't run into a tiger in the parking lot of the supermarket, you are likely to have to deal with a demanding job, an overcrowded schedule, or relationship conflicts. The fight-or-flight response is not an appropriate solution to this type of stressor.

Shelley C. Taylor, at UCLA, has done pioneering work studying a different kind of stress response called tend-and-befriend, which could well be a more important stress response for women than fight-or-flight. She contends that another basic element of the human stress response is the impulse to relate to and work with others. When under threat, people can band together to protect themselves. Our hunter-gatherer ancestors had a clear division of labor: men hunted and women gathered food and cared for children. For women, fight-or-flight might not have been the best defense against predators; young children could be left behind or caregivers compromised by fleeing with young children. The "tend" part of the response was essential for the survival of babies and young children. The "befriend" aspect of the response promotes affiliation. When primitive people worked together as a group, they were more likely to survive.

Humans have developed to use social relationships as a primary resource to deal with stressful situations. Our survival depended on group living. Our ancestors understood that there was strength in numbers and came together to protect themselves and their offspring.

Shelley Taylor discovered that a neuropeptide called oxytocin, which plays a role in sexual arousal, monogamous bonding, childbirth, maternal bonding to newborn, stimulation of milk production, and maternal behavior, is part of an affiliative system that signals the need for social connection. Taylor refers to oxytocin as a "social thermostat" that informs the brain if social resources are adequate to deal with stressful events. Elevated levels of oxytocin may be a biological marker indicating inadequate levels of positive social affiliations.

Oxytocin prompts affiliative behavior when social resources are low. Once positive social contact is established, stress is reduced. If contact with others is hostile or nonsupportive, the stress response is intensified. Just as hunger, thirst, and sexual drives are essential appetites, we need to maintain an adequate level of social relationships that protect and reward us.

## OXYTOCIN AS A MARKER FOR SOCIAL DISTRESS

In 2006, Shelley Taylor and her colleagues conducted a study that measured the psychological and social functions of older women—some on hormone replacement therapy, some not. Oxytocin is enhanced by estrogen. They found that women who had problems in their social relationships had higher levels of oxytocin. These women were more likely to report reduced contact with their mothers, best friends, pets, and social groups. Many had lost their mothers recently, had mothers who were deteriorating physically or psychologically, or had recently lost a pet. Women with high levels of oxytocin did not have a positive relationship with a partner; they viewed their husbands as unsupportive or unaffectionate and felt they could not open up to them.

Several studies found that oxytocin was not related to self-esteem or to general distress. Instead, elevated levels of oxytocin were specifically involved with relationship problems. Another study indicated that elevated oxytocin was associated with anxiety over relationships, coldness, or intrusiveness, and not being involved in a romantic relationship. Shelley Taylor's work demonstrates that social contact and supportive relationships are essential for optimal health and well-being.

The media and popular literature have simplified the role of oxytocin, dubbing it "the cuddle hormone," a natural tranquilizer. That description is inadequate to understand how the tend-and-befriend response actually works. As oxytocin levels rise in response to social distress, we are motivated to seek positive social contact. If positive social contact is made, our stress is reduced. We experience a sense of calm as a result of this positive social interaction. These feelings are likely the result of the effects oxytocin has on two important and specific pathways in your brain, namely the dopamine-reward and the opioid-endorphin pathways. Both of these pathways have motivating and calming effects. This is another example of multiple systems communicating in an integrated and purposeful way to maintain allostasis.

Under acute stress, the oxytocin-dopamine-opioid system can be activated to promote a collaborative tend-and-befriend response, as opposed to a more

### From the Bench

#### THE BIOCHEMISTRY OF FRIENDSHIP

When opioid-blocking medication was given to college students, changes were observed in the women studied but not in the men. The women spent more time alone, spent less time with friends, were less likely to initiate contact with friends, and the interactions they had were less pleasant. This study demonstrates the prominent role that oxytocin and the opioids play in positive affiliative behavior in women—social bonding, initial formation of friendships, maintaining good friendships, and intimate relations.

aggressive fight-or-flight response. Animal and human studies have shown that the fight-or-flight response has to be at least partially inhibited for tend-and-befriend activities to take place. Oxytocin and the opioid pathways have been shown to decrease sympathetic-nervous-system activity and the release of cortisol. The neurocircuitry for social pain actually draws on the neurocircuitry of physical pain—so you really do ache when you are lonely or a relationship ends.

## PUTTING ON THE BRAKES

Not every challenge requires a full-out fight-or-flight/tend-and-befriend response. Social behavior can be stressful, but a subtle shift in perspective might be all that is necessary to adapt. A unique safeguard is built in to your parasympathetic nervous system to keep you from unnecessary arousal and to protect you from the damage of an excitable sympathetic nervous system. That safeguard is called the vagal brake, a concept developed by the pioneering work of Stephen Porges.

The vagus nerve is an intricate neural pathway connecting the brain and the body, including the digestive system and the heart. In 1856, Charles Darwin recognized that the heart and the brain influence each other by means of the vagus mechanism and observed that emotions affect the heart and vagus nerve. In the balanced design of the autonomic nervous system, when the body shifts from sympathetic to parasympathetic, the heart beats faster or more slowly, respectively.

The vagus nerve acts like a brake, slowing down the heart after arousal. The vagal brake is active most of the time to keep the heart from racing and to protect it from allostatic load. When you inhale, the control of the vagal brake weakens and there is an increase in your heart rate. When you exhale, the vagal brake turns back on and your

## Why Tend-and-Befriend Is Predominantly a Female Adaptation

There are real differences between how the sexes relate to others under stress. Oxytocin's effects are strongly enhanced by estrogen, so much so that most research on oxytocin has been done on females. Oxytocin can have stress-reducing effects in men, but testosterone opposes oxytocin, reducing its effect; most men do not have high-enough levels of oxytocin for significant stress-reducing effects. Since women have a stronger affiliative response to stress than men, tend-and-befriend has a more important role in the female stress response, and women have a broad range of relaxation options that are not as effective for men.

heart rate slows down. The difference between these states is called vagal tone. A high vagal tone results in excellent variability even at rest and is an indicator of good health and adaptability to your environment. A chronically low vagal tone indicates little variability and is a reliable indicator of allostatic load. This is a sign that you are less adaptable and resilient to the demands and changes in your environment.

Capable of making minute adjustments, the vagal complex enables us to adapt to threatening events and the emotional and social demands of everyday life. If your response to a stressor is moderate, the sympathetic nervous system does not have to be engaged full-throttle to accomplish your needs. When the vagal brake lets up, an adequate adjustment in heart rate and respiratory function results, without having to engage the fight-or-flight response. Since not everything stressful you encounter in your daily life is an emergency, the vagus nerve allows your body to respond to various levels of stress.

The subtle and elegant adjustments that are permitted by a well-functioning vagal brake allow you to adapt to your complex social world. The vagus nerve influences engagement or withdrawal from the environment. Facial expression, breathing, and vocalization are controlled by the vagal complex. Starting with the communication between mother and child, the vagal system lays the groundwork for the healthy expression of emotions for social interactions. After all, emotion is expressed and communicated by facial muscles.

Since the vagal brake inhibits the sympathetic pathways, it contributes to a state of calm and allows for affiliative behavior.

People whose vagal brake does not function well generally find it more difficult to cope with the demands of the modern world. The proper function of your vagal brake and a healthy parasympathetic nervous system enable you to live in the world, interacting harmoniously with the people and situations you encounter. When you suffer chronic stress, the coordinated actions of the systems we have described are disrupted. That is when your body experiences allostatic load.

## ALLOSTATIC LOAD OR OVERLOAD

Allostatic load is the result of the wear and tear your body experiences as it continually adapts to psychological and physical challenges and adversity.

Many factors affect the regulation of allostasis and account for the differences in individuals' responses to stress. Genetic and early-life adversity definitely play a role in susceptibility to allostatic load. But so do the choices you make on a daily basis. The way you live and even the way you manage your stress contribute to allostatic load. Sleep deprivation, overeating or a rich diet, caffeine and alcohol consumption, lack of regular exercise, prescription or recreational drugs, and anticipation or anxiety can cause internal imbalances that make you more susceptible and less resilient to the effects of chronic stress. These various factors combine to have a direct impact on how your body reacts to stress and can contribute to inefficiency that leads to allostatic load.

Bruce McEwen, who invented the term, described four basic conditions that lead to allostatic load:

- **Too much stress in the form of repeated novel events:**
  If your stress response is activated too frequently, there may not be adequate time for your body to recover fully between periods of arousal. Another possibility with frequent activation is that the response intensifies over time. Remember, this system was designed to be used for quick emergency response, not for frequent activation. In our modern culture, in which stress is often emotional or psychological in nature without a clear beginning and end, this is a common pattern. This condition results from chronically stressful situations, for example, caring for elderly parents, marital conflict, or going through a period of economic hardship.

- **Failure to adapt to the same stressor:**
  If you encounter a stressful situation again and again, you would normally adapt and no longer consider it stressful. With this type of allostatic load, you have failed to adapt, and each exposure is met with the same intense release of cortisol and epinephrine as if it were the first time you were exposed to the stressor.
  Throwing your first dinner party can be extremely stressful. Some women become accomplished hostesses while others are never able to relax and enjoy entertaining even on a modest scale. After a number of tries, you should be able to anticipate and plan a successful occasion. If you still find yourself distraught moments before your guests arrive, you are experiencing this form of allostatic load. No matter how many times you have to do it, you always feel the same and simply cannot be comfortable with it. Perhaps you have never taken steps to become more comfortable.

- **Failure to shut off hormonal stress response after the stressful situation is over:**

  People with this pattern of allostatic load have difficulty in terminating their stress response. Even if their activation is appropriate, they fail to end the response appropriately. The result is that their state of arousal lasts longer than is necessary and becomes detrimental. Genetics and aging contribute to this pattern.

  If there is a history of hypertension in your family, your blood pressure may respond excessively to stress and not return to normal as it should after the stressful event is over. Age also contributes to a slowdown in shutting off the hormonal stress response. With age, the normal mechanisms that are initiated at the onset of the stress response to limit the amount of cortisol produced become less effective. It takes more time for the cortisol levels to return to normal.

- **Inadequate hormonal stress response:**

  This response allows other systems to become overactive. Chronic stress can lead to depletion of stress hormones. Inadequate levels of cortisol affect the immune system and can lead to inflammation and autoimmune disturbances. Under certain circumstances, after chronic or long-term stress, low cortisol may offer some protection despite the alterations in the immune system. Genetic factors and early-life adversity seem to be important determinants of developing this pattern of allostatic load.

As you have seen, the dynamic process of allostasis is constantly at work. Small adjustments in the systems involved are imperceptible. Large shifts, like those necessary to accomplish the stress response, are easily perceived and require activation of balancing systems to prevent allostatic load. Any persistent imbalance between periods of arousal and periods of calm, periods of energy mobilization and periods of energy storage, periods of immune enhancement, and periods of immune suppression will result in allostatic load. The four clinical types that we describe in chapter 4 represent allostasis gone wrong in different ways.

# CHAPTER FOUR

# IDENTIFY YOUR TYPE

## The Four Stress-Response Patterns

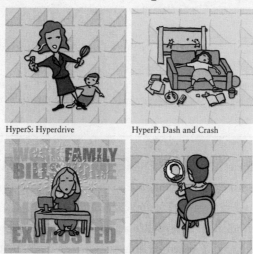

HyperS: Hyperdrive          HyperP: Dash and Crash

HypoS: Fried and Frazzled   HypoP: Detached and Shutdown

A stress response is like a snowflake—no two are the same. Everyone's stress response mobilizes the same core pathways, but there are many differences in the intensity with which we respond and the specifics of how we respond. Your perceptions, genetics, life experience, and your body's health and allostatic systems shape your highly individualized response, as does the nature of the stressor itself, its duration, and the timing of the stress. You would respond differently to each of the following problems: you worked hard for months on a presentation to land a new client and failed; you were responsible

**From the Bench**

Professor Dirk Helhammer, at the University of Trier, in Germany, has identified more than twenty "neuropatterns" that characterize a patient's stress response. This clinical diagnostic and therapeutic tool allows doctors to diagnose where the body's balance gets disrupted and to devise individually tailored care for patients with stress-related illnesses.

Three principles underlie these neuropatterns:

**Ergotropy**—a state of arousal in which the brain and sympathetic nervous system are activated that allows you to adapt to physical or mental stressors.

**Trophotropy**—the opposite state to ergotropy, in which the parasympathetic functions predominate. Sleep, relaxation, regeneration, and recovery characterize this state.

**Glandotropy**—the response of the HPA axis to stress. This refers to the over- or underactivity of cortisol.

Dr. Hellhammer's neuropatterns are an excellent example of bridging the gap between bench and bedside, or using research discoveries to help physicians treat patients.

for a car accident in which you and others were hurt; the head of your child's preschool called to schedule a conference because your son was getting into fights with other children. While some women activate powerful biological reactions to relatively small stressors, others barely move off the baseline when dealing with major events. Some women are simply more stress-sensitive than others. Everyone has a different set point at which the stress response is ignited. **The good news is that you can change your set point to become more stress-resistant.**

## MAKING STRESS PERSONAL

We met with Professor Dirk Hellhammer and his wife, Juliane, at the University of Trier to discuss their groundbreaking work on stress. With the knowledge we gained in our meetings with the Hellhammers, together with our decades of clinical experience and our extensive study of current medical science, we identified four broad patterns of stress responses that we believe can help you. You will be able to recognize your personal type with clues we give you about your habits, behavior, sleep patterns, and medical history. Although Dr. Hellhammer's work actually employs complicated diagnostic tests, assays, and medical histories to make precise medical diagnoses, we designed our more streamlined stress types so that you can recognize yourself and your stress symptoms in them and make changes in your life that will substantially reduce your stress.

## THE FOUR TYPES

Understanding where and how your body tends to go out of balance will enable you to figure out your stress type, and then to select the right techniques that will quiet your stress response and return you to a healthier state. We give specific suggestions for reducing stress with nutrition, exercise, and relaxation techniques in part 2, and full programs in chapter 9, "The Stress-Detox Program for Your Type."

We derived our four stress types by looking at how the HPA axis and autonomic nervous system (your sympathetic [fight-or-flight] and parasympathetic systems [rest-and-restore]) interact under chronic stress. Of course, we are simplifying the very complex reactions your body undergoes when we focus on just these two systems, but they are the core of everyone's stress response.

Here's how your stress response can become overloaded and set you up for health problems:

With **daily hassles,** your sympathetic nervous system is activated and you are in a state of temporary alert, but you can deal with the challenges without distress. Everyday stress doesn't activate the HPA axis with all its messenger chemicals, so your cortisol levels are in your normal range. You may feel tense, irritable, and tired after meeting the challenge, but your health isn't disturbed or damaged.

**Acute or early chronic stress** causes you to experience some amount of distress. Your sympathetic nervous system is engaged and your cortisol levels are elevated. Long-term tension, restlessness, irritability, and exhaustion result. At this stage you can experience sleep disturbances, pain, and gastrointestinal and infectious disorders. Your body can recover from this allostatic load if the stress response is efficiently turned off.

**Chronic or traumatic stress is long-term, persistent distress.** The two systems of your stress response are in gear and working together at either chronically high or chronically low levels, or they dissociate from each other and operate independently. When this happens, cortisol levels can drop, while the activity of the sympathetic nervous system remains high and the pathways that normally restore balance become less effective. Your stress response is out of balance at this stage and your health is affected. This is allostatic load, which becomes destructive in these situations, and anxiety and chronic worry, anger, hostility, depression, sleep disorders, pain, chronic fatigue, weight gain, low libido, high blood pressure, and insulin resistance are common. Autoimmune illnesses can occur.

The progression from the integrated, balanced response that is characteristic of daily hassles to the chaotic disruption in balance and function that occurs with chronic stress happens over time and with repeated exposure to the stress. Since you tend to respond in certain characteristic ways, you may be predisposed to develop specific diseases as a result of chronic, unrelenting stress. Once you are aware of your stress type, however, you can take steps to stop this progression and reverse the effects of allostatic load. Our recommendations are designed to defuse your particular stress response.

The four types we've identified for you as guidelines should be considered a zip code. Identifying your type will allow you to locate a broad area in which you and your stress live. You may find that you have some symptoms from each of the four types, and that your symptoms vary with intensity even within a type. Nonetheless, most of the women we treat do identify with one of the four categories as their primary type. In the near future, we will be able to give you a street address to go along with the zip code for your specific response. In other words, by employing tests like the neuropattern, we hope to be able to narrow down your particular vulnerabilities to a specific location in your body.

For now, we will help you identify your particular stress response among the four basic types.

The four types are:

**HyperS    HyperP**

**HypoS    HypoP**

The illustration below, which resembles a God's Eye, represents the interaction of the two main arms of the stress response. The center of the God's Eye is allostasis, or balance. Chronic stress can push you out of balance and into any one of the types. Within each quadrant or type, you can be close to the center or out to the edge, depending on the intensity of your response and how extreme the allostatic load or imbalance that you've developed. You also can lean more toward one system or the other within the quadrant if either your hormonal system or your nervous system is dominant in your response. This symbol captures the dynamic nature of the stress response and the immense variability in the experience of stress.

## THE FOUR TYPES

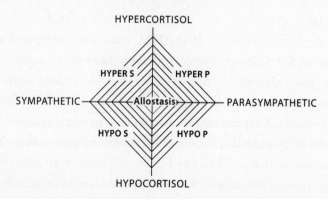

Once you've identified yourself as any one of the types, please remember the icon for your type and record it in your Stress Journal. In part 2, "The Stress-Detox Programs," we advise you about nutrition and exercise and describe various relaxation techniques, the icons at the start of the section will indicate for which types the advice is most relevant. There will also be a Stress-Detox Program for your type at the end of the book.

## THE TYPE ICONS

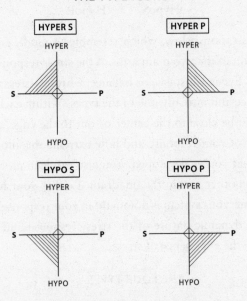

*Hyper* and *hypo* refer to the HPA axis—your hormonal stress system—and the increased or decreased production of cortisol. *S* represents your sympathetic nervous system, which, along with your central nervous system and brain, tends to be activated in the fight-or-flight response. *P* represents parasympathetic (rest-and-restore) activity in the body and a dampening of the central nervous system. These systems normally act in balance, but an overshoot in either direction leads to distress and illness. We will explain how the interaction between the two systems produces emotional, behavioral, and biological symptoms for each stress type.

Symptoms do overlap from one type to another because every stress response utilizes the same messengers and pathways in everyone. The differences are in the communication among the systems activated by stress (sympathetic nervous system and the HPA axis) and the health of the systems that are supposed to help you recover and restore balance (parasympathetic). Yes, just about everyone is tired. But some women are tired because they toss and turn all night, while others never feel rested no matter how much sleep they get. Stress tends to make everyone anxious, but that anxiety can motivate some of us to resolve the problem and others to be debilitated by worry.

As you read the descriptions of the types and consider the symptoms, you will be able to identify groups of behavior, emotions, and physical problems that you tend to experience. We have based our descriptions on findings from the lab bench and our own observations in clinical practice, and we have tried to be as detailed as we can be so that you have a sense of what distinguishes one type from another.

The truth is that very few of us are pure types, but we do have a tendency to react to challenges in a predictable way. Even within a given type your response is individual. Maybe you are susceptible to upper-respiratory or sinus infections, irritable bowel, or lower-back pain. Some of us get colds, others headaches; some of us can't sleep and others can do nothing but. You may feel stress in your stomach, or tension in your neck, shoulders, and back. Perhaps the simple thought of eating nauseates you when you are stressed, or you succumb to stress eating. Even though you probably have some awareness of where and how your body responds to stress, by identifying your general type, you will be able to find the most effective ways to bring your body back to an allostatic state, or balance. Later, in part 2, we explain the right foods, exercises, and relaxation techniques for your type, but here we also provide an immediate tip for each type.

## HyperS TYPE

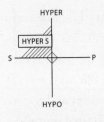

HyperS types have distinct behaviors that make it easy for you to know one when you see one. If you are a HyperS type, you can rarely sit still. You are vigilant, tend to be on edge, anxious, and find it difficult to relax. You are prone to headaches, especially tension headaches, and sinus infections. You often have trouble falling asleep, wake up during the night, and rise early in the morning. Procrastination is not one of your problems, because you consider every task an emergency. You feel you must complete your work as quickly as you can. You are a multitasker. You can be short with words, because you are eager to keep moving forward. Your communication is direct and to the point. Though you can become exhausted from lack of sleep and from driving yourself to expend great amounts of energy, you may become more wound up and frantic as your exhaustion progresses. You can be emotional, expressive, and, at times, explosive.

## THE ELEMENTS OF A HyperS RESPONSE

A HyperS response occurs when the classic fight-or-flight response is activated too frequently or does not turn off properly. The demands and challenges of daily life stimulate this response. HyperSs are usually high-functioning. The main characteristic of this type is the constant arousal of the brain and the sympathetic nervous system. Your body is on alert, so the HPA axis is activated, and cortisol levels are high. One of the primary functions of the activated HPA axis is to make sure the brain is supplied with glucose, the energy it needs during this time. In this hypervigilant state, brain function is focused to evaluate and respond to the stress.

## Real Life

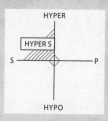

Charlene, at forty-two, was suffering from severe headaches. She was anxious and having difficulty sleeping.
Already thin, she had lost fifteen pounds. She asked
Stephanie to prescribe sleeping pills for a few nights. She
was given a prescription for a small number of pills and
cautioned about their long-term use. The medication really
didn't help. She returned, certain that she was seriously ill. Stephanie scheduled a
battery of tests—a full blood work-up and an MRI of her brain. All the tests were
normal.

In the course of the appointments, Stephanie learned that Charlene had recently
returned to work. She had been very successful selling medical equipment, doing
an outstanding job in a competitive industry, but had stopped working when her
first child was born, and now had three children, ages nine, ten, and eleven. She
had loved being a full-time mother, had been active at the children's school and in
the community, and she enjoyed entertaining. Her husband had worked in finance,
but he had lost his job when the economy crashed. Suddenly, their entire situation
changed: Charlene had to contribute to the family income to keep the home they
loved. She wanted to find work locally to be near the kids, but a decent job was
not available. Charlene was rehired by her old company. Her symptoms had begun
during the uncertain time before her husband lost his job and intensified after she'd
gone back to work.

Although Charlene had always been active, busy, and social, her reaction to her
family's financial pressures had triggered an acute stress response that she could
not shut off. It was classic fight-or-flight gone wrong. If she had not changed her
life to relieve the pressure, she would have continued on her way to becoming seriously ill. After several conversations with Stephanie, Charlene realized that she
could not keep up the pace of her life and the pressure had to give somewhere. She
and her husband decided to sell their home and to rent instead. Her husband found
a job that would cover their expenses, and she was able to cut back on her hours.
Her symptoms resolved quickly, and she began to gain back the weight she had
lost.

With HyperS types, the key element of the imbalance is that your
sympathetic nervous system has put your entire system into overdrive.
This can occur if oxytocin and other pathways are unable to balance
the norepinephrine release in the brain in response to stress or if serotonin and other calming pathways are weak and unable to restore

balance. You can think of this state as the brain being unable to quiet itself. This is allostasic load. Nerves trump hormones in the HyperS response.

Your body is not meant to be in this overexcited state for long. It mobilizes too much energy and overtakes your metabolic, immune, and central nervous systems. If you activate this highly charged system too frequently or are unable to turn off this response effectively, you will get sick. HyperS women develop stress-related diseases more than any other type.

High cortisol levels and the sympathetic-nervous-system overdrive contribute to changes in carbohydrate and fat metabolism. You store and concentrate fat around your middle and you become insulin resistant. Cortisol also has effects on the cardiovascular system that can lead to heart disease and arteriosclerosis, or hardening of the arteries. Cortisol directly alters the immune system, which is why HyperS women catch colds easily. The accompanying sympathetic overdrive also contributes to high blood pressure, rapid heart rate, sleep disturbances, and agitation.

Below is a list of typical behaviors and complaints of women with HyperS tendencies:

- Restlessness/over-activity
- Tapping fingers and feet/ leg shaking
- Nervousness
- Nail biting
- Grinding teeth
- Quick talking
- Plagued by time and deadlines
- Always on time
- Fear
- Increased vigilance
- Anxiety
- Trouble sleeping
- Irritability
- Change in memory
- Excessive exercise
- Tension in shoulders and neck
- Headaches

- Loss of appetite
- Acne
- Flushing of skin
- Increased sweating
- Nervous stomach/irregular bowel function
- May be lean but tend to gain weight in the abdomen

- Tends to go to bed and rise early
- Palpitations
- Change in menstrual cycle
- Decreased libido

---

### Real Life

Julie was home for Christmas break from her first year at an Ivy League school in the East. She came to see Stephanie because she had stopped getting her period. Stephanie talked to her about life at college.

Julie was surprised that she was having such a tough time adjusting. She found the workload daunting and felt much less sophisticated than her classmates, many of whom had known each other for years from eastern prep schools. She was working all the time and felt that building new friendships was a luxury she couldn't afford. She had taken to going to the gym to work out at ten o'clock most nights to get an energy boost so that she could squeeze in a few more hours of study before turning in, averaging no more than five hours of sleep a night.

The food on campus was awful—it was hard to find the local fruits and vegetables she was used to eating in Southern California. Now a size 0, she was happy to be losing weight, but Stephanie suspected that Julie was developing an eating disorder—all the symptoms were there. Stephanie recommended that Julie bring her mother in so they could talk about the way Julie was feeling and recommended that Julie seek treatment for her developing eating disorder through a center at her school. She advised Julie to move her exercise regimen to the morning and to do some of her exercise outdoors when the weather permitted. They discussed nutrition, though the specifics of this would also be addressed by the center at her school. She advised Julie to make a specific point to seek out friends, because some of what was causing Julie to feel poorly was social isolation. In her second year of school, with changes in places and an awareness of her stress-response tendencies, Julie was able to adjust and began to thrive and enjoy her college experience.

If nothing is done to bring the body into balance, HyperS types are likely to develop:

- Cold sores
- Frequent colds
- Panic disorder
- Anxiety disorders
- Obsessive/compulsive disorder
- Chronic sleep disorders
- Alcoholism
- Other addictive behavior
- Bladder infections
- Yeast infections
- Ulcers
- Depression
- Anorexia nervosa
- High blood pressure
- Heart disease
- Osteoporosis
- Type 2 diabetes
- Sexual dysfunction
- Infertility/amenorrhea

### Do you see yourself?

1. Are you a fidgety person?
2. Do you grind your teeth?
3. Do you find it hard to eat when you are under stress?
4. Do you have trouble falling asleep?
5. Do you wake up in the middle of the night and worry about the next day?
6. Do you respond to everything with anxiety?
7. Are you forgetting things?
8. Do you get stress headaches?
9. Do you have a nervous stomach?
10. Do you need to exercise intensely to burn up nervous energy?
11. Do you get colds all the time?
12. Are you prone to addictions?
13. Even if you are thin, do you tend to gain weight around your middle?
14. Are you an early riser?

## HypoS TYPE

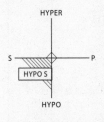

HypoS symptoms are less obvious than those of a HyperS type. You can become anxious and fearful when stressed and are more likely to hide out or retreat under pressure. Women with a HypoS response tend to be calm, but even a little stress can provoke a big response. Your type is extremely stress-sensitive.

A triad of symptoms is associated with this type: fatigue, pain, and increased stress sensitivity. As a HypoS, you often feel as if you never get enough sleep. You tend to develop food allergies and hives. You often have unexplained aches and pains, and you wonder after a while if they are all in your head. You go from doctor to doctor looking for answers, often with little success. Nevertheless, the pain is real. You have pain in your back, pelvis, bladder, or vulvar areas.

You often lack the energy for multitasking and describe yourself as exhausted or drained. HypoS types tend to be overweight, but you do not have as much cortisol-induced weight gain around the middle as the HyperS type has. Your weight gain tends to be more in your hips and thighs. You have less trouble sleeping than a HyperS, but you don't wake up refreshed. You tend to stay up late and have trouble getting out of bed in the morning.

## THE ELEMENTS OF HypoS

In the chronic stress response of HypoS, the HPA axis and the sympathetic nervous system are not in sync. They have dissociated. The HPA axis is either unable to produce enough cortisol or the normal, healthy daily rhythm of cortisol production has been lost. In a normal stress response, cortisol helps to balance and modulate the stimulated nervous system. When the cortisol effects are inadequate, the already-

## Real Life

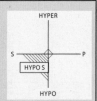

Tracy had recently moved to Southern California with her husband, because he had an extraordinary job offer in a start-up firm. At twenty-nine, she had left a career she loved as an associate editor at a fashion magazine; she missed the excitement of putting out a magazine each month and the glamour of a world she had inhabited since college. She had left her friends, family, and countless contacts, and the notion of establishing a network of support in Southern California seemed daunting. She just didn't have the energy to follow up on some leads with friends of friends to figure out something to do that would challenge her creatively.

She was having trouble getting out of bed in the morning and still hadn't gotten around to doing more than unpacking the cartons in their new place. Her asthma, which hadn't troubled her since college, was acting up again. Hungry all the time, craving foods that had never touched her lips, she was concerned that she was depressed. When Tracy confided in her mother, her mother told her that she had gone through a stressful time when she was pregnant with Tracy. Tracy's father was transferred overseas and her mother had to manage most of the move by herself. Just as they were getting settled, Tracy's grandmother became seriously ill, and her mother flew back and forth from Europe to the States as often as she could. Though the pregnancy itself was smooth going, Tracy's mother said it had occurred at the most difficult time of her life. She encouraged Tracy to enjoy the California sun and to get outside and exercise. When Tracy told Beth this story, Beth thought there might be a connection between the difficulties in Tracy's mother's life while she was carrying Tracy and Tracy's stress response and stress sensitivity.

Tracy tried, but just couldn't muster the get-up-and-go. She ached all over and couldn't focus long enough even to finish reading a magazine article. She made an appointment with Beth, because she had begun to have unbearable pain with sex. Each time she and her husband attempted intimacy, she had to grit her teeth just to get through the act. Pleasure was not even the goal for her at that point—all she wanted was to get through it without extreme pain.

She looked normal on physical examination, but the pelvic exam was very painful for her, something that had never happened to her before. We began treatment for a condition called vulvodynia, which involves a hypersensitivity to the nerves in the skin of the vulva. No medication provided any relief.

Since friction had begun to grow in Tracy's marriage, Beth suggested that Tracy and her husband get relationship counseling, because vulvodynia is very tough on a marriage. After several months of visits to Beth, however, Tracy stopped coming back, and Beth didn't see her again for a year.

When she returned for her annual checkup, Tracy was a different person—smiling and radiant. She and her husband had decided to split. Even though their relationship had always been tumultuous, Tracy had hoped that moving with him to the West Coast would change things, but it hadn't worked out. After they'd separated, Tracy got back to keeping her lithe, fashionista body in shape, which had led her to start a new career as a Pilates instructor. This had opened up a whole circle of friends, and she now had a new boyfriend and had been having sex comfortably since they'd met.

aroused brain and sympathetic nervous system can overreact. Because the production of norepinephrine in the brain is high, the sympathetic nervous system also remains revved up.

Cortisol keeps your immune function in check, so low levels of cortisol take the brakes off the immune system. This can result in an overactive immune response that attacks the tissues of your body, resulting in arthritis, thyroid problems, lupus, increased inflammation, asthma, and pain sensitivity.

Research has shown that experiencing in utero stress or early-life adversity can alter brain anatomy and brain sensitivity to stress hormones and shape this sort of stress response. In addition, in-utero stress may directly limit the capacity of the adrenal glands to produce cortisol in response to the stress signals from the brain.

HypoS women are at risk for developing a broad range of diseases. The media have given attention to the damaging effects of stress-induced high cortisol levels, and, as a result, some people believe that hypercortisolemia—the overproduction of cortisol—is the most damaging imbalance. You might think, therefore, that low cortisol levels would have health benefits, but this is not necessarily the case. It appears that low levels of cortisol occur in susceptible people when they have been exposed to chronic stress over long periods of time. Some researchers believe that this drop in cortisol production is an allostatic effort by the body to protect itself from the damaging effects of high cortisol, but that this adjustment overshoots in the opposite direction and leads to a different type of allostatic load. This primarily involves an overactive immune system and leads to pain and fatigue and a central nervous system that is too easily stimulated. The HypoS type overadjusts, limits the effectiveness of the HPA axis, and unleashes the sympathetic nervous system.

Please look at the list below to see if you have had any of these symptoms, tendencies, or past experiences in times of stress:

**Real Life**

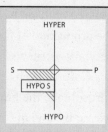

Sharon, a longtime patient, had come to the office for a routine visit. During the pelvic exam, Stephanie noticed that Sharon appeared to have developed genital warts, a sexually transmitted infection. Sharon had recently celebrated her twenty-fifth wedding anniversary. When Stephanie told her that she had a sexually transmitted infection and needed a biopsy, Sharon was visibly shaken by the news.

When the biopsy confirmed the diagnosis, Sharon was confronted by the fact that her husband had been unfaithful, most likely during his frequent business trips. Sharon was thrown into a confusing emotional state—terrified to leave her husband and start all over in her fifties and furious with her husband for betraying her. Filled with self-doubt as well as rage, she became weepy, anxious, and irritable. She didn't want anyone to know what was going on, particularly their two children away at college. When she confronted her husband, he was contrite and suggested that they have marital counseling.

Sharon became exhausted and ached all over. She began craving comfort food and put on weight. She blamed herself for what she was going through, because she couldn't bring herself to end her marriage even though she felt it was permanently broken. The conflict was painful on every level. When Stephanie saw Sharon again, she diagnosed her with autoimmune thyroid disease. The thyroid is particularly vulnerable to stress, and women over forty have a relatively high incidence of thyroid disorders, but Sharon's condition was treatable with medication. Sharon went into therapy, resolved to save her marriage, and worked with Stephanie to create a stress-detox program to restore her health and build her resilience. She is still dealing with marital conflict, but her health remains improved.

- Early life adversity, including in-utero maternal stress
- Extreme stress sensitivity
- Inability to concentrate
- Increased sleep
- Late to bed and difficulty getting up in the morning
- Increased appetite
- Muscle tension
- Fatigue/exhaustion
- Chronic pain
- Lack of motivation, inactivity
- Shakiness
- Blood pressure fluctuations
- Gastrointestinal complaints—nausea, diarrhea, vomiting

- High body mass index with a propensity to gain weight in the hips and thighs
- Increased susceptibility to inflammation

This list of diseases that HypoS types are likely to develop demonstrates that low cortisol can be as damaging as high cortisol levels:

- Seasonal depression
- Postpartum depression
- Chronic fatigue syndrome
- Eczema, seborrhea, psoriasis
- Panic disorder
- Low-back pain
- Chronic pelvic pain
- Fibromyalgia
- Premenstrual syndrome
- Interstitial cystitis (inflamed bladder)
- Allergies
- Asthma
- Heart disease
- Autoimmune thyroid disorders
- Lupus
- Irritable bowel syndrome
- Rheumatoid arthritis
- Osteoporosis
- ADHD
- Chronic vulvar irritation or pain
- Post-traumatic stress syndrome

### Do You See Yourself?

1. Was your mother's life very difficult or stressful during her pregnancy with you?
2. Were you a premature, low-birth-weight infant?
3. Did you have early adversity in your childhood, such as malnutrition, divorce or death of parents, frequent moves?
4. Do little things that don't bother other people stress you out and seem too hard to deal with?
5. Are you exhausted?
6. Are you troubled by general aches and pains?

7. Do you eat emotionally for comfort?
8. Is just the thought of exercising enough to make you tired?
9. Do you have a hard time getting up in the morning?
10. Do you have eczema, psoriasis, or hypersensitive skin?
11. Do you have severe PMS?
12. Do you have lower-back pain?
13. Do you have allergies or asthma?
14. Do you have seasonal depression?

## HypoP TYPE

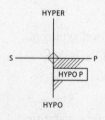

HypoP is the rarest stress response, an extreme state caused by a severe imbalance. If you are a HypoP type, you often feel as if you are a spectator in your own life. You tend to be detached from the world, and withdrawn, as you do not feel stimulated by people and the world around you. You may get dizzy when you stand up suddenly, and you faint easily. Extremely sensitive to stress, you feel helpless and tend to be passive when dealing with adversity. You may have difficulty expressing your feelings. In fact, your feelings may seem buried so deeply that you cannot gain access to them. You rarely express either pleasure or emotional pain. You do not smile often and tend to speak in a flat, expressionless tone. You often have aches and pains and even get abdominal cramping in emotional situations, but you do not make the connection between the physical and emotional.

## THE ELEMENTS OF HypoP

The HypoP stress response results when the HPA axis, the producer of your stress hormone, cortisol, and sympathetic nervous system,

## Real Life

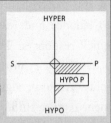

Lori and her husband, Tom, are very close. Tom is everything to Lori, and he never disappoints her. One day, while working in his vegetable garden, Tom doubled over with horrible chest pain. Carrying a glass of iced tea out to the garden for Tom, Lori found him lying on the ground, holding his chest. She called 911 and comforted him until the ambulance came.He had a heart attack that required a long period of recuperation. Suddenly, at forty-two, Lori had to be responsible for running their lives and caring for the man she loved so much.

At first, she welcomed the concern of friends and family, but she became too exhausted to deal with visitors. Though she appreciated their concern for Tom, she was incapable of talking about her own feelings. Every phone call, email, and drop-in began to seem like an imposition. She was having a hard time staying on top of all that had to be done and resented anything that distracted her from taking care of Tom and creating a serene environment for him. She didn't want to talk or even think about the heart attack and how close she had come to losing her husband. But even though she didn't want to worry Tom and tried to be cheerful around him, she had begun to feel that she was close to the limit of how much she had to give— and felt as if she were looking at her life through a thick fog. When she wasn't with Tom in the bedroom, she would sit staring into space, feeling helpless and alone. She often forgot to eat and was having abdominal cramps and dizziness.

When her mother flew in from the Midwest to help, she was more distressed by Lori's condition than Tom's. Lori had always been self-effacing and somewhat withdrawn, but her detachment had become much more severe. Her mother insisted that Lori see a doctor, convincing her that she had to take care of herself or she wouldn't be able to help her sick husband. When Lori came in to see Beth, Beth suspected that she was a a HypoP stress responder.

Beth suggested that Lori begin to keep a journal of her emotions, especially when she was having disturbing physical conditions like abdominal cramping. She recommended specific nutritional intervention to help control Lori's immune response and give her more energy. She also had Lori begin to exercise slowly and with low impact. When Lori was able to give herself a little more attention and make changes, she began to recover. The following year, Lori's husband had recovered from his heart condition and Lori was feeling much more like herself again.

the arouser of the body for challenge, are in sync but functioning at chronically low levels. This might seem desirable, because it means your body is not in a hyperaroused state, but it actually represents a severe imbalance. HypoPs are dominated by the effects of the parasympathetic nervous system—the system that is meant to balance and restore you after the sympathetic nervous system's quick responses. The dynamics of this stress response are complex; a deficiency in norepinephrine production in the brain is one possibility. Arousal, vigilance, and active participation with the environment require sufficient levels of norepinephrine. A HypoP imbalance drains you of vitality and joy. Your abnormal cortisol levels throughout the day affect your immune functions, metabolism, and blood pressure.

The gastrointestinal tract is particularly vulnerable to stress in the HypoP type because of the increased parasympathetic activity. This system is in control of our digestive functions. The combination of the low cortisol and increased parasympathetic activity make even small adjustments difficult for HypoPs. The routine day-to-day demands on the HPA axis, brain, and sympathetic nervous system can be a burden for the suppressed energy of the HypoP type.

The symptoms of a HypoP response are pronounced because they are extreme:

- In-utero/early-life adversity
- Fatigue/exhaustion
- Withdrawal from people and activities
- Lack of drive or motivation
- Boredom
- Learned helplessness
- Decreased sweating
- Increased stress sensitivity
- Slow heart rate
- No energy
- Passive behavior
- Poor muscle tone
- Tendency to black out or faint
- Abdominal cramping
- Diarrhea
- Drop in blood pressure with minimal alcohol use
- Tendency to feel light-headed when standing up too quickly

## Real Life

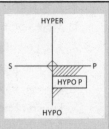

Juliette sat slightly slumped on the examination table, looking listless. She told Stephanie that her boyfriend had insisted she come for a checkup, because she had nearly fainted the other day when she got up from the conference table at work after a long meeting. She had resisted her boyfriend's suggestion to make an appointment with Stephanie, insisting that she was just tired.

When Stephanie asked her what was wrong, she mumbled that she was always exhausted and had lost interest in just about everything. She was suffering from stomach cramps and diarrhea, and everything seemed to stress her out. Though Juliette's boyfriend had filled Stephanie in prior to the appointment, Stephanie was surprised to find her patient so drained. Juliette had always been extremely reserved, and Stephanie had suspected that Juliette had had some severe problems in the past. During her conversation with Juliette's boyfriend, Stephanie learned that Juliette was isolated without any close friends and had begun to avoid all social contact.

As they talked during the examination, Stephanie learned that Juliette's boss and mentor had left the company for a big position elsewhere and had been replaced by a tyrant whose expectations were unpredictable and unrealistic. Juliette was having a hard time adjusting to the demands of her new boss, who kept calling attention to her and was never satisfied. She just didn't know how to please him. Everyone at the office had been affected, and the tone of the place had changed from warm and trusting to harsh and edgy. Juliette knew she was not handling it well at all. After several months, it was making her sick.

Stephanie explained to Juliette what kind of stress reaction she was having, that she was a HypoP type. She recommended that she begin with exercise in the early morning, a Pilates video with a very slow introduction to the program, and recommended that she go to bed early and use melatonin to help her sleep pattern. She also had Juliette make specific dietary changes to give her energy and an improved rhythm in her cortisol production. At her follow-up visit, though her working environment was still not ideal, she admitted to having more energy and feeling more upbeat.

Aside from a miserable quality of life, HypoP women are at risk for developing:

- Asthma
- Ulcerative colitis
- Inflammatory disorders
- Learned helplessness

### *Do You See Yourself?*

1. Were you a premature baby?
2. Are you extremely exhausted?
3. Do you lack drive or motivation?
4. Do you tend to be passive?
5. Do you find yourself withdrawing from people?
6. Are you bored?
7. Do you have trouble expressing your feelings?
8. Do you experience abdominal cramping and diarrhea when you are stressed?
9. Do you have poor muscle tone?
10. Does just a little bit of alcohol affect you strongly?
11. Do you often feel faint or light-headed?

# HyperP TYPE

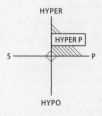

HyperPs are likely to be high achievers who go, go, go until they collapse like a fallen soufflé. Even on a weekend or a vacation, when a HyperP woman has time to relax, she tends to overshoot: instead of reaching a balanced state, her nervous system goes from being in high gear to crashing. You are spent, drained, and barely able to function when you melt down. You spend some Saturdays on the couch with slight nausea and blurred vision. After adequate rest, you usually bounce back to normal.

With HyperPs, symptoms occur after the stressful situation has passed. Your response is a dramatic shift from overdrive to collapse. Although many feel this way at the end of a busy day, the HyperP response is extreme, and recovery from it requires more than just vegging out. You need to retreat or withdraw for at least one to four days before your balance is restored.

## THE ELEMENTS OF HyperP

HyperP is a transient state that occurs after your stress is permanently or temporarily relieved. You may feel profound fatigue, altered mood, and a lack of initiative and motivation. This occurs when the norepinephrine supply in the brain has been depleted by prolonged periods of overdrive and vigilance. The parasympathetic, or restoration, system becomes temporarily dominant. You feel extremely exhausted and find it difficult to maintain focus and concentration. The HPA axis functions normally in response to stress, but the two arms of the stress response—the hormones and nervous system—are temporarily out of sync until the norepinephrine levels are replenished.

**Real Life**

Elaine is a prominent trial lawyer in her fifties, admired by friends and family for being able to do it all—marriage, children, a busy practice, demanding trial work, involvement in charities, an active social life—and to look terrific while juggling so much. She seemed to thrive on stress.

At her annual checkup, she told Stephanie of a pattern that had emerged over several years. When she went on family vacations and had a chance to relax, she would become a different person—exhausted, withdrawn, and quiet. She wanted to sleep rather than ski, snorkel, or hike with the family. It was as if she crashed and burned as soon as she stepped off the daily treadmill. She was so effective at maintaining a state of high gear in her regular life that the moment she had a chance to relax, she collapsed. Her family was hurt by this repeated pattern; they felt as though she had time for everyone else, but when she was away with them she needed to be alone. After a few days she would recover from her stupor and reengage with her family with renewed energy, but she felt as if she had to make up for her collapse, and that started the cycle over.

With Stephanie's advice, Elaine began to start her vacation a day or two before the rest of the family. Either she would go away early or take a time off before her vacation to unwind. This enabled her to enjoy every day of vacation with her family. They also discussed what she could change in her life to avoid collapsing in the future.

With rest, calm, and adequate protein consumption, your norepinephrine stores come back efficiently and you recover to allostasis quickly. However, if a HyperP goes too long in this state, we suspect that she can progress to the more severe state of HypoP. This is clinical conjecture on our part. But all the signs and symptoms indicate that HyperPs are candidates for burnout.

The transient symptoms for HyperPs are:

- Extreme exhaustion
- Inability to do anything
- No energy
- Listlessness
- Irritability
- Overemotional
- Need for sleep

- Withdrawal
- Poor concentration
- Exercise intolerance
- Feeling faint
- Nausea
- Prone to dehydration
- Blurry vision

---

### Real Life

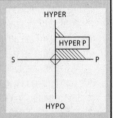

Julia, forty-one, has two children ages nine and eleven. Twice a month, her husband would organize a special Saturday with the children so that Julia could have some time alone to pamper herself or be with her friends, without the kids. He became concerned, though, when her idea of a day off was to climb into bed and pull the covers over her head. He was sure that she was depressed or that her hormones were imbalanced, and he encouraged Julia to make an appointment. When she saw Beth, Julia said that her episodes of extreme exhaustion were not cyclic and had nothing to do with her monthly cycles. She was juggling a lot—they were renovating the kitchen, so she was living in a construction site; the children played sports, so she was running them to practices and games; and they had a new puppy, who was very demanding. Overwhelmed and anxious, she was having difficulty sleeping and had no desire to eat even if her kitchen had been in working order.

Julia explained that, while she did it all, the prospect of an extended break with nothing she needed to do caused her to let it all go and collapse. By the time her family returned at the end of the day, she was restored and happy to hear about their adventures. Beth explained that her collapses were a stress response that she could avoid by following the HyperP Stress-Detox Program, described in chapter 9.

Given proper rest on a regular basis, you will return to allostasis and will not develop disease states. If you do not restore yourself, you are at risk of developing:

- Ulcers
- Performance incompetence
- Progressive, profound fatigue
- Lack of motivation

- Inability to initiate new activities
- Burnout
- Decreased libido

### Do You See Yourself?

1. Are you a major multitasker?
2. Do you have boundless energy—until you stop?
3. Do you seriously crash some weekends?
4. Do you shut out the world when you collapse?
5. Do you ever spend all of Saturday or Sunday in bed or fail to leave the couch?
6. Do you need to be isolated to restore yourself?
7. Do you always get sick the first few days of vacation?
8. Do you find any demands on you overwhelming when you are in this state?
9. Are you irritable?
10. Is your vision blurry?

Whether you are a HyperS, HypoS, HyperP, HypoP, or some combination, you have to understand that these states are not static. They are snapshots of your characteristic response to stress, but not full portraits. These four types represent the primary manifestations of stress that we see every day, and they are mutable. As chronic stress progresses or when it becomes unrelenting, you can move from one type to another. If you are a HyperS and your adrenal glands become burned out from long-term stress, you can become a HypoS. If you are a HyperS and your norepinephrine stores become depleted, you can become a HyperP. We believe that HyperPs are at risk for burnout of cortisol production, which could move you to a HypoS or HypoP. We think it unlikely, however, for a HypoS or a HypoP to become a HyperS or HyperP.

Whether you identify wholly with one type or recognize yourself in all four, what's important is that you understand how your mind and body are vulnerable to stress and affected by it. Now you are in a position to begin to undo the destructive impact of chronic stress. Part 2 of *The Ultimate Stress-Relief Plan for Women* will give you the tools you need to manage your stress and restore your equilibrium, vitality, and pleasure.

# PART TWO

# THE STRESS-DETOX PROGRAMS

CHAPTER FIVE

# THE FOUNDATIONS OF STRESS RELIEF

## Relaxation, Restorative Sleep, and Natural Rhythms

Now, as you are beginning to read this chapter, take a survey of your body. Can you drop your shoulders? If you can, you are holding more tension in your muscles than you should be. Is your brow furrowed in concentration? Are you holding this book tightly, clenching your jaw, or grinding your teeth? Are you perched on the edge of your chair? Your posture and the way you hold yourself indicate the degree of tension you are experiencing, but they can also actually elicit a stress response; tense muscles send a message to your brain that stimulates the cerebral cortex, which then arouses the HPA axis, your hormonal alarm system, and the autonomic nervous system, which is responsible for your protection and survival. Whether you are tense because you are stressed or stressed because you are tense, taking a moment to loosen up your body will make a big difference.

When you are stressed, your body can assume an aggressive or defensive posture. The way you stand—pitched forward or back, chest out or shoulders slumped—often reflects your appraisal of a situation or your view of your place in the world. Just as muscle tension can be a sign of psychological stress, holding tense postures can create stress.

Gripping, clenching, and tightening your muscles prepares you to escape or to attack but can cause fatigue and pain as well. Muscle tension and immobility can stress your joints and reduce your blood flow, contributing to decreased energy and feelings of fatigue and strain. Tension headaches, neck and shoulder pain, and a bad back often develop as a result of how you hold yourself. If you have tense muscles, you are also more likely to worry and to stay upset longer.

Notice the way you are breathing. Is it shallow, from the top of your lungs? Is your diaphragm involved, causing your stomach to move in and out, or are you relying on the muscles of your rib cage and shoulders? Are your breaths rapid and uneven? When you are calm, your breath should be even and full, which can help you relax. This type of breathing can reduce your heart rate and depress the activity of cortisol, the major stress hormone. When breath is rapid and shallow, carbon dioxide levels in your blood can change and can lead to feelings of dizziness, anxiety, and panic. Stressed breathing uses more energy and stimulates all your internal systems and processes indiscriminately.

Are you able to concentrate on the words on the page, or do you find yourself focusing on stiff joints, a nervous stomach, or other things going on in your body? Are you considering how tired you are or how much you have to do later? Do those thoughts make you anxious, depressed, or angry? Where your mind wanders can be a good indication of the nagging concerns that are fueling a stressed state in your body. Sometimes, just thinking about a condition can aggravate the symptoms.

Taking stock of how tense and distracted you are at this moment can give you a sense of your level of stress. You might feel as if you are reasonably relaxed and your attention is focused on reading, yet, when you observe yourself objectively, you find residual signs of the day's stress in your body. Stress can be such an integral part of your life that you might become accustomed to physical and emotional tension and lose touch with what it feels like to be relaxed and open. In this part of the book, we want to show you why it is so important to take stock regularly of how you are feeling so that you can begin to undo the long-term effects stress has had on your body and your life. No matter which of the four stress types you are, we will show you in the following chapters how to move back to center, balancing your body's systems to restore your energy, vitality, health, and happiness. Many of the recommendations we will make apply to all four stress types. As we go, we will highlight those that are especially effective for each particular type, so that as you read, you will see your plan unfolding.

Reducing stress is a highly individualized process. What works for you might not work for your best friend. Your idea of relaxation may differ from hers, too. You might want to manage your stress, enhance your sleep, or encourage healing. You might want to boost your energy or good health in order to be able to take action calmly, to be more productive and effective. Perhaps you want to increase your creativity, enjoyment, or understanding. Or your goals might be transcendent, inspiring mindfulness and spirituality. Whatever your goals, we'll provide a variety of tactics that you can try in order to reduce your stress.

When your body is out of sync, allostasis is disrupted and you are more susceptible to the physical and emotional effects of stress. But when your multiple internal systems are well coordinated to maintain allostasis, you thrive. This is the fundamental principle we want you to understand as you begin to make lifestyle changes.

Making these life changes means you are taking responsibility for your health. This can be frightening. Many people ask their doctors for a magic pill that will rid them of their symptoms and make them better. Most of us would rather be diagnosed with a recognized illness that has a set treatment than have to confront complex symptoms

**Real Life**

Renee, a dynamic woman of sixty-one, looked as if she was in her forties. She was a successful interior decorator whose work was getting a lot of attention. She was turning away business from all over the country, because she was just too busy and in such high demand. When she came to see Stephanie for her annual exam, she was regularly commuting to Aspen to oversee work on a mogul's ski lodge. She had been getting increasingly exhausted and was beginning to notice more aches and pains, especially in her neck.

Renee had rarely had any physical problems. In fact, she had flown through menopause without serious symptoms, although she takes a low dosage of hormone replacement therapy to extend the protective effects of estrogen on her mind and mood. At her annual checkup, however, both she and Stephanie were shocked to discover that Renee's blood pressure was a high 150/92 (normal is generally 120/70. Stephanie suspected that Renee was a HypoS stress responder—her sympathetic nervous system was in overdrive without an opportunity to rest and recover, so her blood pressure was elevated.

Since Renee wanted to avoid a lifelong dependency on medication, Stephanie suggested that they take one step at a time, eliminating possible solutions that did not work. They started with the easiest—meditation. Renee had no trouble focusing, and she could meditate on planes, in cars, and in hotel rooms. Motivated to bring down her blood pressure, she changed her diet, meditated twice a day for a total of forty minutes, and increased her daily walks. Her blood pressure was under control within two months. Even better, meditation brought a lot to her life: she felt more balanced and rooted and attained a level of relaxation that rejuvenated her and allowed more creative thoughts into her life and work. She credited meditation with lifting her creativity to new levels.

that have no prescribed course for relief. It seems easier to take a pill than to change your life by developing healthier habits and creating balance.

We are not saying that you are responsible for getting ill. And we are definitely not saying that you have failed if you cannot control a disease you've contracted. Having read about the complex interactions of the systems within you, you probably have an appreciation of the many things you simply cannot control. What we want you to take away from this book is a sense of what you can do to improve your health and well-being. We especially want to teach you how to protect yourself from the chronic stress that will eventually wear you down.

## Relaxation

Although the importance of relaxation has been recognized since ancient times, Herbert Benson, a Harvard University cardiologist and director of the Mind/Body Medical Institute at Harvard, made a significant breakthrough in the early 1970s. His studies revealed that we have an innate ability to reduce our heart rate, blood pressure, and brain-wave activity, a self-protective process he calls the "relaxation response." The response, a mirror image of the stress response, employs the parasympathetic system—the rest-and-restore system—to reduce arousal.

When he studied practitioners of Transcendental Meditation, Benson found that, during meditation, subjects dramatically decreased their heart rate, breathing rate, blood pressure, and metabolic rate; these physical changes suggested deepening relaxation. **Benson and his colleagues theorized that, just as the fight-or-flight response could be triggered by many different stressors, methods other than Transcendental Meditation would produce the relaxation response.** The researchers found that it didn't matter if you sat or stood, were quiet or chanted. There were countless ways to achieve the relaxation response—through yoga, walking, swimming, gardening, basically any activity that took you out of yourself. Research showed that the relaxation response was an effective way to treat headaches, premenstrual syndrome, anxiety, and all but profound depression.

The expanding research of Benson and his colleagues revealed the powerful connection between mind and body. The work they published in medical journals was controversial because it challenged the accepted notions of traditional Western medicine that the body's physical systems were unaffected by emotions or conscious mental processes, which they believed were unmeasurable. More than thirty years later, Benson still pursues the scientific study of the relaxation response as well as nutrition, exercise, and stress management.

**From the Bench**

**HERBERT BENSON AND THE RELAXATION RESPONSE**

In the latest edition of *The Relaxation Response,* Benson writes:
"One by one, we have identified medical conditions that can be relieved or altogether eliminated with the help of the Relaxation Response, remembered wellness, and other self-care approaches. . . . We learned that, with self-care, we can effectively treat any disorder to the extent that it is caused by stress or mind/body interactions. Indeed, we can partly relieve or cure most of the common complaints patients bring to their doctors' offices simply by applying self-care techniques. By taking advantage of the cost-free, healing resources within all of us, the United States, by conservative estimates, stands to save more than $50 billion in wasted health care expenditures each year."

Benson lists conditions that he and his colleagues have found to improve significantly or heal by the use of self-care techniques:

- Chest pain
- Irregular heartbeat
- Allergic skin reactions
- Anxiety
- Mild and moderate depression
- Bronchial asthma
- Herpes simplex
- Cough
- Constipation
- Diabetes mellitus
- Duodenal ulcers
- Fatigue
- Hypertension
- Infertility
- Insomnia
- Nausea and vomiting during pregnancy

- Nervousness
- All forms of pain, even postoperative
- Premenstrual syndrome
- Rheumatoid arthritis

Benson's decades of work with thousands of patients and study participants have demonstrated that all illnesses have a mind/body component and could potentially be helped by the use of relaxation techniques. Did you notice that his list shows diseases and symptoms that span all four stress types? Learning how to invoke the relaxation response will benefit you no matter what your stress type is, but you can also derive specific benefits for your particular type.

**HyperS:** You have high cortisol production and an overactive sympathetic nervous system, which makes you feel anxious and agitated. Relaxation lowers your blood pressure and anxiety. It slows you down, improves your sleep. You can use relaxation techniques to help you avoid or overcome dependencies and addictions.

**HypoS:** You are very stress-sensitive, because your sympathetic nervous system is unchecked, and your low cortisol level also leads to overactive immune reactions. You are prone to inflamed joints and muscles and have low energy. Relaxation will calm you and protect you from your tendency to have extreme reactions to stress. It will help you to combat your fatigue, your pain, and your discomfort.

**HypoP:** You are withdrawn and your systems are in shutdown. Your cortisol levels are low and your parasympathetic nervous system is dominant. Relaxation will help give you the space and perspective to cope with others. Learning how to relax will enhance your physical health and help you to connect with your emotions as you learn to identify when your physical symptoms arise as the result of suppressed emotion. Relaxation can also rebalance your sympathetic and parasympathetic nervous systems.

**HyperP:** You are in overdrive and your cortisol production is high, but your sympathetic nervous system is so charged up that it can become depleted of its major neurotransmitter, norepinephrine. Daily use of relaxation techniques can help you to restore your burned-out energy and prevent your periodic crashes.

## RELAXATION GOALS

Herbert Benson studies a general physiological process that can be set off by many different sorts of relaxation. More-recent approaches to relaxation focus more specifically on physical parts of the body as well as on a number of more defined psychological states. Jonathan C. Smith, a clinical psychologist and director of the Roosevelt University Stress Institute, believes that relaxation creates more than physical stress relief and has shown that stress management does far more than simply reduce your heart rate: the experience of relaxation affects your perception and experience of the world.

Learning and mastering a stress-defusing technique takes only about a month, but if you stick with it, you will increase the long-term benefits to your health and longevity. The emotional and mental states that you can experience from relaxation can also be rewarding in and of themselves. When you practice restoration techniques as part of your life, you can change and grow in ways you would not expect.

Jonathan C. Smith studied the descriptions that thousands of peo-

**From the Bench**

**THE CYCLE OF RENEWAL**

"All relaxation evokes a fundamental process of healing and growth in which one withdraws from the efforts of the day, recovers, and opens up to the world. I call this the Cycle of Renewal. The ideal of a cyclical renewal process has been around for several millennia and can be manifest at many levels. World religions speak of global cycles of death and rebirth, repentance and forgiveness, as well as acceptance and enlightenment. Professional approaches to relaxation involve mastering the discipline of withdrawing from everyday stress for healing and recovery, and returning to the world refreshed and restored. And each time we pause and sigh we display a moment of relaxation and renewal."

—From Jonathan C. Smith's book ABC Relaxation Theory.

ple gave of their relaxation responses and organized them into twelve basic feelings:

- Physically relaxed
- At ease/peaceful (mentally relaxed)
- Sleepy
- Accepting (giving up control)
- Aware/focused/clear
- Disengaged (feeling removed, distant, neutral)
- Optimistic
- Joyful
- Mystery (experiencing insight into profound meaning)
- Quiet (still mind/no thought)
- Reverent/prayerful
- Timeless/boundless/infinite/at one

When you're relaxed, you can experience a variety of states that are distinct and beneficial. The twelve different feelings or outcomes can give you a better idea of what you want from your relaxation practice.

Which of the above states would be a goal or goals for you? You might want to make a note in your Stress Journal.

Smith described four categories of relaxation and renewal in this way:

**Basic relaxation** involves reducing your physiological arousal or revved-up state so that you can feel physically relaxed, disengaged from any worries, sleepy, peaceful, and at ease. HyperPs and HyperSs in particular live in such a charged-up state that they have to achieve basic relaxation before they can be open to experience other states of relaxation. HyposSs need to maintain a state of calm as their response to stress is so exaggerated.

**Core mindfulness** is the essential element of many relaxation techniques. Focusing on the world around you and blocking out your constant stream of stress-inducing thoughts helps you to achieve feelings of awareness, focus, clarity, quiet, and acceptance. Core mindfulness is an important goal for HyperSs, because you are chronically preoccupied with stressful thoughts and perceived challenges.

**Positive energy** is a state in which you are aware of beauty, harmony, happiness, and humor. Joy and optimism are directly related to your health and longevity. Positive energy is a particularly good goal for HypoPs and HypoSs, who need a boost to regain your overall vitality.

**Transcendence** is the recognition of something greater than yourself and a feeling of connection to it, whether you experience God or the grandeur of the universe. In this state, you will feel reverent/prayerful/mystery/infinite/or at one with everything. Every stress type would benefit from being in this elevated state.

According to Smith, the process of renewal and reversing the powerful impact of stress occurs in three stages. First, you withdraw from the world, mentally. Then you begin the recovery stage, in which you let go of your stress and feel relieved. Finally, you open yourself up again to receive fulfilling and positive energy from the world within and around you. Regardless of what you choose to do for relaxation, you will go through these same three stages in the process.

To achieve the positive feelings that Smith describes, you have to dedicate a small amount of time each day to relaxation. Practice the techniques that you eventually select so that they become a habit. Just as you would not leave your house in the morning without brushing your teeth, we want you to think of your relaxation as important to your health and appearance as basic hygiene. In fact, you should consider relaxation a basic hygiene practice for your health.

## NATURAL RHYTHMS AND RESTORATIVE SLEEP

Learning how to relax has a powerful effect on our patients, and the results are even more dramatic when they have improved their health with restorative sleep and have synchronized their bodies to natural rhythms. Stress disturbs the rhythm of your body. This is because your body's natural daily rhythm, called "circadian rhythm," is largely synchronized by the stress hormone cortisol. Stress disrupts your cortisol production in different ways for each of the four stress types. If you are a HyperS or a HyperP, your inherent rhythm of cortisol production is maintained, but you have strong surges within those cycles that result in high levels of cortisol. If you are a HypoS or a HypoP, however, your natural rhythm of cortisol production is lost and your cortisol levels are lower, so that when you experience stress you are still able to produce a small burst of cortisol, but your brain and body overreact. Restful sleep, proper nutrition, regular exercise, and the daily practice of restoration techniques will readjust your inner clock and help to restore your body to balance.

For maximum stress resistance, you also need an adequate amount of restorative sleep. And to get high-quality sleep, your biological clock needs to be in sync with the twenty-four-hour natural rhythm, the amount of time it takes the earth to rotate on its axis, that regulates all life on our planet.

## THE CLOCK WITHIN

Your body has an internal clock, a daily biological or circadian rhythm that regulates your active and rest states with biochemical reactions that are synchronized to the day's hourly, light–dark cycle. The role of the circadian clock is to promote wakefulness during the day and sleep at night. The period of the human sleep/wake cycle is longer and more variable from day to day than the biorhythms of most other animals, and your body takes cues from the environment, such as light, temperature, food, and activity level around you, that synchronize or entrain your internal rhythms to the earth's twenty-four-hour rotation. Light has the most powerful effect on your internal clock.

Your stress response type has a big impact on your circadian rhythm, so we will make recommendations specific to each stress type on how to balance your system and prevent disease by synchronizing your circadian rhythm.

You achieve the best sleep when you are in sync with the natural cycle of light and dark, because all of your allostatic pathways are responsive to these inherent rhythms. Peaks in cortisol during the day are associated with wakefulness, and declines are associated with sleepiness. If your cortisol pulsing is strong and exaggerated, as in the HyperS and HyperP types, you may rise abruptly and early and have difficulty falling asleep. You also awaken often during the night and have trouble going back to sleep. Restful sleep is a cornerstone to recovery from stress-system disorders, so we will give you many suggestions in the coming chapters to help decrease cortisol production for the HyperS and HyperP types. If you are a HypoP or a HypoS, eating your meals on a predictable schedule, regular exercise, and consistent times for sleeping and awakening will regulate the natural rhythm of cortisol production and get you back on track to allostasis and health.

## LARKS AND OWLS AND THE FOUR TYPES OF STRESS

"Morning" people, called larks, wake up early and spring to life, and "night" people, or owls, stay up until the wee hours of morning and sleep late whenever possible. We believe that HyperS and HyperP types are more likely to be larks, because of their strong cortisol peaks that promote early awakening and provide them energy in the morning.

Melatonin, a neuropeptide produced in the brain, also contributes to the regulation of your circadian rhythm. Melatonin produces sleepiness by communicating with the brain pathways that promote sleep. You can use it as a supplement to help entrain your circadian rhythm with the natural cycles of light and dark where you live. But please do not think of melatonin as a sleeping pill. When taken in the evening, melatonin sets the body for nighttime and helps you to fall asleep and awaken earlier. Taken in the morning, melatonin causes you to fall asleep later at night and awaken later. The use of melatonin to change sleep and wake times works best if you take melatonin at a specific time each day. In fact, it may be harmful to take it at varying times, because it can promote desynchronization of your inner clock. The effects of melatonin supplementation are greatest after several weeks of use. You may feel drowsy when you first use it as a supplement, and the lasting beneficial effects take time to develop. Two to three weeks of use are necessary for entrainment of your circadian ryhthm.

## LARKS, THE EARLY RISERS

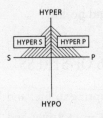

If you are a lark, like the HyperS and HyperP types, your biological clock is set several hours earlier than that of the average person. You tend to fall asleep between 6:00 and 9:00 p.m. and wake between 2:00 and 5:00 a.m. You become extremely sleepy in the late afternoon or early evening. As you get older, regardless of your stress type, your clock is likely to shift in this direction.

### What to Do If You Are a Lark

- The most effective way to synchronize your rhythm is to expose yourself to bright artificial light in the evenings, which will delay your early-evening pulse of melatonin production. This can improve sleep quality and increase total sleep time.

- Just two days of light exposure in the evening has been shown to improve sleep and cognitive performance in adults with early-morning insomnia.

- If you would like to shift your rhythm, you could try to go to bed thirty minutes later every two days until you reach your desired bedtime.

## OWLS, LATE TO BED AND LATE TO RISE

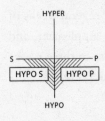

If you have trouble falling asleep before 2:00 to 5:00 a.m. and prefer to wake between 10:00 a.m. and 1:00 p.m., you are an owl and most likely a HypoS or HypoP. Sleeping late decreases your exposure to early-morning light and that can promote more late sleeping. Staying up late, and especially being in bright, artificial light delays the production of melatonin. Owls are more sensitive to evening light. This rhythm is more common in adolescents regardless of their stress type. As any mother knows, trying

## Real Life

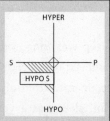

Rebecca, age nineteen, confessed to Stephanie that she was worried that she had a sleep disorder because she could never fall asleep until well after midnight. She was fine if she could get eight hours' sleep and didn't have to be up until midafternoon, but she had problems with morning classes. To Rebecca's embarrassment, she had nodded off in several classes. She also complained of feeling unusually fatigued even when she did get enough rest. Her mother was concerned by her lack of energy. Checking her chart, Stephanie noticed that several members of Rebecca's family had rheumatoid arthritis, an autoimmune disorder. Stephanie suspected that Rebecca might be a HypoS type.

Since Rebecca was in college, she could keep to her natural rhythm since it worked for her body. She could choose classes later in the morning or in the afternoon. But what would happen after she graduated and got a job? Stephanie explained circadian rhythms and advised Rebecca to use exercise in the mornings, to eat her meals at consistent times during the day, to expose herself to bright light in the early mornings, and to avoid bright light in the late evenings to entrain her rhythm to be earlier. She also recommended using melatonin in the evenings. After two to three weeks of following this advice, Rebecca's clock began to reset.

to get a teenager out of bed on a Saturday morning can be a serious challenge after the night owl has been up until early morning listening to music or playing video games.

## What to Do If You Are an Owl

- Take 0.3 to 3mg of melatonin five hours before bedtime for three weeks.
- Avoid bright light in the evening and dim the lights after dark.
- Expose yourself to one to three hours of bright light between 7:00 and 10 a.m.
- Try to go to bed fifteen to thirty minutes earlier every two or three days until you reach your desired bedtime.

When your circadian rhythm is desynchronized and you are deprived of sleep, every system in your body undergoes significant physical stress.

## SLEEP IS A DYNAMIC STATE

Sleep was long considered by scientists to be a passive state. Many believed that sleep's purpose was simply to give the body a chance to recuperate from all the energy expended during the day. As it turns out, sleep has a very different, dynamic purpose in your life. Sleep helps you to process emotions, retain memories, and relieve stress. We want you to understand how this happens. Many important changes occur in your body and mind every night as you sleep.

There are five well-defined phases of sleep. A good night's sleep has about five cycles of these phases and requires approximately eight hours to complete the process.

**Stage 1:** This is a drowsy state that lasts for five or ten minutes. Your eyes move slowly under your eyelids, and your muscle activity slows down, but you are easily awakened. You might experience sudden muscle contractions, jerky movements that resemble the startle reaction we make when we are surprised.

**Stage 2:** During this stage of light sleep of about twenty minutes, your eye movements stop, your heart rate slows, and your body temperature decreases. Your brain waves slow except for an occasional burst of rapid waves called "sleep spindles."

**Stage 3:** With this thirty-to-forty-minute stage of deep sleep, blood flow to the brain decreases and is redirected to your muscles, allowing restoration of your cells. Immune functions decrease during deep sleep. Theta and delta waves, which are slow brain waves, synchronize at this phase, and the number of sleep spindles lessens. Restorative sleep begins with this stage.

**Stage 4:** This deep stage also lasts thirty to forty minutes, and it is very difficult to awaken from. You are groggy and disoriented if aroused from this or the preceding stage. Your brain gives off delta waves, the slowest brain waves. Your breathing and heart rate are at their lowest levels in the cycle. This is the most restorative stage of sleep.

**REM Sleep (Dream Sleep):** About seventy to ninety minutes into each cycle, you shift into REM sleep, during which your blood pressure and heart rate rise. Your eyes dart around under your eyelids. Your brain waves are similar to those when you are awake. Your breath becomes shallow, rapid, and irregular. If you wake up during REM sleep, you might remember strange stories that are outside normal logic. These are your dreams. Your body is essentially paralyzed during REM sleep, perhaps to keep you from acting out your dreams.

Once you have gone through the five stages of sleep, the entire cycle repeats itself. All night long your brain cycles between complex stages of lower and higher activity, from deep, restorative sleep to more-alert stages and dreaming. **Deep sleep is the most critical stage of sleep.** When you are sleep deprived, your brain will spend more time in deep sleep and less time in the other phases, so, to help yourself recover from sleep deprivation, you should go to bed earlier. Non-REM sleep prevails in the first stages of sleep, but as the night progresses, REM-sleep stages increase in length and your sleep becomes lighter. When your deep-sleep cycles are interrupted or cut short, you will feel the effects of sleep deprivation most powerfully. REM sleep helps to boost your mood during the day. **If you want to improve your mood, allow yourself to sleep a little more in the morning, when REM sleep is longer. Sleeping an extra half hour can be a big help.**

Several studies have shown that a nap during the afternoon restores wakefulness and improves performance and learning. One study found that a short daytime nap reduced levels of anger and augmented joy and relaxation, improving the mental states of the subjects after the nap. If you nap for thirty minutes or less, you do not reach stage 4, REM sleep. Recent studies have found that frequent long naps may actually have long-term, adverse health consequences because they affect the quality of your sleep at night and disrupt your circadian rhythm. It is preferable to get your sleep at night. A cat nap during the day can be refreshing, just don't overdo it.

In the course of a normal night, you will spend 20 percent in deep, slow-wave sleep, 25 percent in REM sleep, 50 percent in non-REM sleep, and 5 percent awake. This balance changes as we age. After sixty, people tend to spend only 5 to 10 percent of their night in slow-wave sleep, 10 to 15 percent in REM sleep, and they can be awake as much as 30 percent. Completing all five cycles of sleep is essential for your brain to deal effectively with stress. Restorative sleep allows you to resolve allostatic load and sharpens your mind to face the challenges of a new day. Too little sleep or sleep that is interrupted is stressful for your brain. Getting restorative sleep is the essential first step in combating the effects of stress.

## A TIME OF SLEEP DEPRIVATION

Even though no one would deny that she needs quality sleep to be healthy, upbeat, and energetic, adults and adolescents have been sleeping one and a half to two hours less a night for the last fifty years. People are working longer hours into the night, playing or working on computers, or doing chores late at night they didn't have time for earlier.

Surveys conducted by the National Sleep Foundation reveal that at least 40 million Americans suffer from sleep disorders. Sixty percent of adults report having sleep problems, including difficulty falling or staying asleep, early awakening, and interrupted, nonrestorative sleep a few nights a week or more.

## SLEEP DEPRIVATION AND YOUR WEIGHT

The trend toward shorter sleep times has happened at the same time as a national increase in obesity and diabetes. Research has found that partial sleep loss is linked to obesity and diabetes, and it clearly disrupts key components of appetite regulation and changes your carbohydrate metabolism. Between 2000 and 2006 there were ten published studies that consistently reported an association between not getting enough sleep and high body mass index in adults. These studies, conducted in Spain, France, Germany, Switzerland, and the United States, revealed that sleep loss increases the risk of obesity.

Not getting enough sleep also has a direct effect on your appetite. The chemicals and hormones that play a role in controlling appetite and weight gain are released during sleep. Since leptin, an appetite suppressant, is produced at night, the amount you sleep affects how much is produced. Ghrelin, a peptide released in the stomach that increases your appetite, is normally produced before meals to stimulate your appetite. When you are sleep deprived, your leptin levels go down while your ghrelin levels increase, which means you are hungrier and therefore inclined to eat more.

### From the Bench

#### LEPTIN, GHRELIN, AND SLEEP DEPRIVATION

One thousand men and women kept sleep diaries, recording how many hours they slept each night. Each subject spent one night sleeping in a laboratory. A blood sample was drawn the next morning. The researchers found that having a typical sleep time of five hours as compared with eight was associated with leptin (a hormone that suppresses appetite) levels that were 18 percent lower and ghrelin (a peptide that increases appetite) levels 15 percent higher—a perfect storm for weight gain.

## MELATONIN AND WEIGHT GAIN

Melatonin is directly involved with weight regulation and energy balance. Melatonin, produced at night, is a complex hormone involved with body weight, energy balance, and sleep in humans. The duration of melatonin production is related to the length of the dark phase of each day. Light suppresses the production of melatonin. Since days are shorter and nights are longer in winter, you produce more melatonin in the winter months. The prolonged production of melatonin during the winter months is associated with weight loss. Conversely, the longer hours of daylight in the summer months result in shorter periods of melatonin production and weight gain. In cold-weather climates, you may see weight gain in the winter, because you are more sedentary. In climates where you can be active year round, you may notice weight gain in the summer, a result of the effect of melatonin on your metabolism. It is a mechanism your body uses to store fat for a cold winter. All types will notice this shift in their metabolism seasonally. Taking melatonin in the summer may help boost your metabolism. You could try a small dose of 2 to 3 mg in the early evening around 5:00 or 6:00 p.m. on the long summer days.

## SLEEP AND THE HPA AXIS

According to George P. Chrousos, a prominent stress researcher, insomnia isn't just a nighttime problem, it is a disorder of emotional and physiological hyperarousal that is present day and night. Under normal circumstances, sleep, deep sleep in particular, inhibits the two major arms of your stress system, the HPA axis and the sympathetic nervous system, and prevents a state of constant arousal and vigilance. When sleep is disrupted, you lose allostatic balance.

Even though insomniacs complain about their daytime fatigue, they tend to be significantly more alert than normal sleepers. This is because insomniacs' brains and bodies are revved up around the clock. This condition of twenty-four-hour, stress-related hyperarousal of both the brain and the autonomic nervous system is characteristic of the HyperS type. If you suffer from insomnia, you have a higher heart rate, decreased circulation, and increased musculoskeletal movements when you are awake *and* when you sleep. Your vagal brake is not functioning properly. You also show faster brain-wave patterns than normal sleepers at every stage. Your brain metabolism stays elevated even when you do get to sleep. Since your nervous system stays on, shifting from wakefulness to sleep is difficult.

Cortisol, which is overproduced in HyperS and HyperP types, increases your brain waves and stimulates wakefulness. It also decreases your REM sleep and increases your time spent awake during the night. High levels of cortisol in the evening, when cortisol is normally declining, can explain why you might awaken a number of times each night. Higher evening levels of cortisol can also be seen with HypoS and HypoP types due to the overall disruption in their cortisol rhythm. In a twenty-four-hour study, ACTH and cortisol levels were significantly higher in insomniacs compared to normal sleepers. The greatest elevation occurred in the evening and the first half of the night, when cortisol levels should drop. The higher the coritsol level, the greater the amount of sleep disturbance experienced.

## A HEALTH WARNING ABOUT FREQUENT INSOMNIA

If you experience insomnia three or four times a week for a month, you should get help. If insomnia is triggered by specific external stressors and lasts a month, the condition is known as "transient insomnia" and is usually resolved once you adjust to the stressful events that are causing you sleep problems. If the symptoms last six months or more, you are suffering from chronic insomnia.

We want to make you aware of other issues that are associated

### Real Life

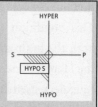

Genevieve, age fifty-eight, was concerned about her weight, which was inexorably inching up. She had gained ten pounds in the last few months, although her hormones had seemed to have reached a steady state. She had always eaten carefully, but now found herself hungry all the time. Exercise had always been part of her life, but she felt she needed to do more to stop her weight gain, and she asked Stephanie for advice.

Stephanie knew that Genevieve took good care of herself. She wasn't sedentary or eating fast food. She answered that she had been having a hard time getting to sleep at night and would toss and turn for hours. She was working on complex projections at the office, and her boss was micromanaging her work, which was counterproductive. She had spoken to him and tried to keep it professional, but he had been so wound up that he erupted. Ever since, she felt she could not be open with him. His stress had been contagious. She felt as if the project would never end.

Stephanie believed that Genevieve was a mild HypoS stress responder and that this was affecting her sleep, which was influencing her weight gain. Genevieve was surprised to hear that there was a connection, but realized that her weight gain coincided with the start of the project.

Stephanie explained how Genevieve could use light to entrain her circadian rhythm, making it easier for her to fall asleep earlier, and suggested that she move her exercise outdoors. The timing of Genevieve's exposure to light could affect her sleep. Stephanie suggested that she get light exposure in the morning and dim the lights prior to her bedtime. Stephanie also recommended that Genevieve set aside a time each day to think about the friction at work and to focus on making it better, suggesting that midday would be the optimal time, so that it was distant from bedtime. She advised Genevieve to keep a journal about her conflicts with her boss. Recording what happened, how she felt, and how she handled the situation would help to clear her negative emotions and give her insights into the problem.

Genevieve incorporated Stephanie's suggestions into her routine, and although she was not able to influence her boss, she began to sleep better, and the end of the project was in sight. In three months, her weight had returned to normal.

with insomnia. Women experience insomnia more often than men. Menopause is one explanation for the differences in sleep disturbances between middle-aged women and men. One study of menopausal women found that the amount of time it takes to fall asleep increased in postmenopausal women who were not on hormone replacement therapy. Those women were less likely to have stages 3 and 4 sleep as well. The increased prevalence of depression in women is another reason we tend to experience insomnia more than men do. Insomnia occurs more often in women who are separated, divorced, or widowed.

People with a lower economic status and those who are unemployed are more likely to have sleep problems. Aging is also a factor associated with insomnia, which affects 50 percent of people over sixty-five. Some personality characteristics can predispose you to insomnia, namely depressed mood, rumination, chronic anxiety, inhibition of emotions, and inability to express anger.

The abnormal changes in the daily rhythm of cortisol secretion in the HypoS and HypoP types cause specific sleep problems. Low cortisol levels can limit your ability to cycle normally through the stages of sleep, leading to lower-quality sleep. You may sleep for eight or nine hours at night but not feel refreshed when you wake up in the morning. You may also find it harder to get up and go in the mornings because of low levels at the time of day you should have a peak level.

Not only is lack of sleep dangerous to individual health, but it has been connected to international disasters such as the *Exxon Valdez*, Chernobyl, Three Mile Island, and the *Challenger* shuttle explosion, as well as the hundred thousand traffic accidents a year that occur because of driver fatigue, which result in fifteen hundred fatalities.

### Some of the Many Benefits of Sleep
- Allows the brain to organize memories, solidify learning, and improve concentration
- Helps to maintain innovative and flexible thinking
- Regulates mood
- Affects social interactions and decision making
- Affects motor skills
- Strengthens immune system
- Regulates carbohydrate metabolism, which keeps you from putting on weight
- Allows rest-and-repair in nervous system
- Replenishes energy stores in brain cells needed to repair cellular damage caused by an active metabolism

- Growth hormone released during sleep repairs muscles
- Contributes to cardiovascular health

## HOW MUCH SLEEP DO YOU NEED? AND CAN YOU MAKE UP FOR LOST SLEEP?

The amount of sleep you require is regulated by a brain mechanism called the "sleep thermostat." The homeostatic process works by increasing your tendency to fall asleep in direct proportion to the increasing size of your sleep debt. The size of your sleep debt determines how strong your urge to fall asleep becomes.

Adults, in general, need seven to eight hours of sleep to be healthy, although some can get by with five hours and others require ten. Women in their first three months of pregnancy need more than a solid eight hours. It is not true that older people need less sleep: although you sleep more lightly for shorter periods as you age, you still require the same seven or eight hours. Exactly how much sleep you need depends on your age, genetics, and what you do when you are awake. If you stand on your feet all day, do hard physical labor, or are training for a triathlon, you will probably need more sleep than someone who sits at a desk eight hours a day.

There are a few signs you should look for to gauge whether you are sleep deprived. Do you need to nap often? Do you have what sleep researchers call "microsleeps," brief episodes of sleep during the day when you just drop off for a moment? Do you fall asleep within minutes of going to bed? Do you need an alarm clock to wake you in the morning? If your answer is yes to any of these questions, you very likely need to change your habits and get more sleep.

You have to make up for lost sleep to stay healthy and productive. After a bad night or two, say you are working long hours to meet a deadline, you just need to sleep longer for the next couple of days. **We don't recommend routinely cutting down on sleep during the week**

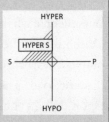

**Real Life**

Elizabeth is a spunky, cheerful eighty-five-year old who is always a delight when she comes in for her exams. But she seemed troubled at her most recent yearly exam. Her son had been offered a terrific job and was moving three thousand miles away with his family. They wanted her to move with them, but she was reluctant to leave the home in which she had lived for more than fifty years. She had lost her husband ten years ago and now lived alone in the house they had shared. Her other children had relocated. Only one granddaughter remained in town. She was worried about what to do. She still had many friends in town, but found she was turning down invitations to lunch and was not making it to social events at church. She was napping more and found that she was unable to sleep more than three hours at a time at night. Though she made up for the sleep loss during the day with catnaps, she was finding it more and more difficult to sleep at night. As a consequence, she was not getting enough deep sleep to restore herself.

Beth advised her to increase her activity during the day. She suggested that when Elizabeth felt sleepy, she should take a walk instead of a nap. Beth encouraged her to spend more time with her friends and family. Increasing her activity during the day would help reset her biological clock.

Elizabeth gave it a try, and three months later, she was sleeping more consistently through the night. This gave her renewed energy and clarity in dealing with her decision to remain in her home, and her granddaughter became more active in helping to care for her.

and sleeping in on the weekend. If this becomes a habit, you could disrupt the overall quality of your sleep and incur more-serious long-term side effects. If you have had long-term sleep deprivation—maybe you have a baby or are taking care of someone who is recuperating from surgery—you should try to catch up every few days. Try to sleep as long as you need to during this payback period. Your body will return to its optimal sleep pattern.

## SHIFT-WORK SLEEP DISORDER

Regardless of your type, this advice applies to you if you do not work the traditional hours of nine to five. If you work night shifts or swing shifts, you need to know how to maximize your restful sleep. Twenty percent of the workforce of industrial nations work nonstandard hours. People whose jobs require them to work through the night and to sleep during the day can develop chronic sleep deprivation and a complete desynchronization of the systems of their bodies, leading to allostatic load. The severity of shift-work disorder depends on age, responsibilities at home, commuting times, type of work schedule, and the worker's natural circadian-rhythm tendencies. Since shift workers

---

**Real Life**

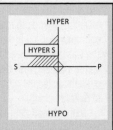

Tanya, a thirty-six-year old homemaker, is a lark and a HyperS stress responder. Her body demands that she go to bed early, and she wakes up as the sun rises no matter how much she wants to stay asleep. She is sleepy in the evenings but pushes past these feelings to get ready for the next day. After the children are in bed, she prepares lunch, snacks, and uniforms for the following day for her three children. When she finishes those chores, she watches TV with her husband. She always falls asleep on the couch and has to be awakened by her husband to go to bed at 11:30. Every morning she wakes up at 5:00 a.m. regardless of how well she slept. She lies in bed until 7:00 trying to fall back to sleep.

Beth recommended that Tanya watch TV with her husband after the children went to bed and then turn in early. Beth suggested that when Tanya wakes up at dawn, she should get up and do the preparation for her children's day. Shifting her schedule this way would fit with her body's natural rhythm.

---

often have to work and sleep at times in opposition to their circadian rhythm, their alertness can be severely compromised. Shift work is associated with increased depression, alcohol or drug abuse, gastrointestinal symptoms, sleep apnea, obesity, and miscarriage.

## WHAT TO DO ABOUT JET LAG

Jet lag disrupts your biological rhythms. If you travel regularly, no matter what your stress-response type, you need to pay attention to entraining your bio-rhythm to make you more stress-resilient. Jet lag is characterized by daytime sleepiness and fatigue, insomnia, mood changes, difficulty concentrating, general malaise, and gastrointestinal problems. The direction in which you are traveling and the number of time zones you pass through influence the severity of your jet lag, because your body's rhythms are out of sync with the local time. To

---

### What to Do If You Work Shifts

- Have caffeine at the beginning of the shift.
- During the night shift, get bright light continuously or intermittently during the first half but then, if possible, dim the lights for the last two hours of the shift.
- If you work the night shift, wear sunglasses during the ride home in the morning light.
- Take 3 mg of melatonin three hours before bedtime.
- Use eye covers and block out light from windows to help you sleep during the day.
- Use earplugs so that you are not disturbed by daytime noise.
- Keep the room as cool as it would be at night, because temperature affects circadian rhythm as well.

---

minimize jet lag, wear loose clothes when traveling, and drink fluids, but avoid caffeinated and alcoholic beverages or food during the flight to avoid travel fatigue. Do your best to eat meals at local times, to exercise, and to stay awake while there is daylight at your destination.

Strategic exposure to light can help you reduce the effects of jet leg or avoid it altogether. East-bound travelers should expose themselves to bright light in the early morning and dim the lights in the evening. If you are going west, expose yourself to sunlight in the late afternoon and evening and try to stay awake until it gets dark.

## HOW TO GET A GOOD NIGHT'S SLEEP

There are many factors in modern life that can interfere with your ability to get a good night's sleep. Caffeine, diet pills, and decongestants can stimulate parts of your brain that cause insomnia, and many antidepressants suppress REM sleep. Smoking can also cause you to sleep lightly with reduced REM-stage sleep; people who smoke tend to wake up three or four hours after falling asleep because they experience nicotine withdrawal. Alcohol can help you fall into a light sleep from which you are easily awakened, but it interferes with REM and deeper sleep. Studies have shown that middle age and menopause make you more susceptible to sleep disturbances, particularly since your sensitivity to stimulating substances like caffeine is intensified. Long-term use of sleeping pills produces no clear-cut health benefits and may shorten your life span. Sleeping pills may work for a short-term problem, but they should be avoided as a long-term solution.

Here is a list of helpful tips for changing your lifestyle that will help you sleep better. They are useful to all four stress types:

- Do not smoke, especially near bedtime or if you wake up in the night.
- Avoid alcohol and heavy meals before sleep.
- Get regular exercise, but not within a few hours of bedtime.
- Employ stress-management techniques in the course of your day.
- Do not nap during the day if naps make sleeping at night more difficult.
- Go to bed and wake up the same time every day, including weekends, even if you don't get enough sleep. Observing a schedule will train your body to sleep at night.
- Make certain your bedroom is quiet, dark, and cool. If you

cannot control the noise, use a fan, earplugs, or a white-noise machine.

- If you have to sleep during the day, use an eye mask and hang blackout shades on the windows.
- Have a bedtime routine and do the same thing every night before going to sleep. You might read, take a bubble bath, or have a glass of warm milk. Milk contains tryptophan, which stimulates the production of serotonin, which in turn plays a role in inducing sleep. A cup of chamomile tea is also helpful before bed. It increases the release of a neurotransmitter called GABA, which calms you. Your mind will connect these activities with sleep, and observing the routine will eventually make you sleepy.
- Use the bedroom only for sleeping or having sex. Avoid intense conversation, watching TV, or talking on the phone in bed.
- Do not lie in bed worrying about things. Set aside another time—perhaps after dinner—to think about what you can do about what is worrying you. Writing your concerns and potential solutions in your Stress Journal can be helpful.
- If you remain awake after trying to sleep for thirty minutes, get up and go to another room. Sit quietly for approximately twenty minutes before going back to bed. Do this for as long as it takes you to fall asleep.

## THE LAST RESORT: STRESS AND MEDICATION

As physicians with an active clinical practice, we know that there is sometimes a need for medications that deal with the very real and, at times, incapacitating physical and emotional complaints of our patients. The use of these medications must be part of an individualized, comprehensive care plan for each patient. Each medication can be helpful and yet still have side effects that you might find intolerable or that themselves require additional medication to manage. If medication seems a critical part of your treatment, you will have a better response to the medication and may require lower doses by incorpo-

**Real Life**

Laura, in her late thirties, was single and lived alone. She was a very popular hairstylist, and her calendar was always overbooked. The pace of her work was more demanding than she wanted. She went out with girlfriends from the salon often, but did not feel close to them. She usually had several drinks when she went out, and she started having difficulty sleeping.

Laura had moved to California from the Midwest and missed her family. She longed for a steady life with a husband and children, but hadn't met the man for her. Worrying that she might not have children, she had become anxious and depressed. She began to take Effexor, which was prescribed by her internist. Although she felt less anxious with the medication, she also felt emotionally flat and began to gain weight, even though she had not changed her exercise or eating habits. After six months of exercising more and eating less, her weight was up, not down. She decided that she would rather be anxious than fat and stopped her medication abruptly. She immediately felt as if she had the flu and was nauseated, exhausted, and lethargic.

During her annual gynecologic exam the next day, Laura told Stephanie what was going on. Stephanie explained that Laura should not stop that kind of medication abruptly and was feeling ill because she had not used her medication for the past two days. She told her to restart at a lower dose and recommended a safe way to taper off. Relieving worry and stress is not as simple as taking medication, and Stephanie explained that if Laura did not make lifestyle adjustments, she would most likely require more and more medication and would then have to deal with yet more side effects and possibly less-beneficial effects over time. Stephanie encouraged Laura to make dietary changes that would improve her sleep, including eating food at breakfast and not simply drinking a large cup of coffee as her morning meal, to cut back on her alcohol consumption, start her day with exercise, expand her social network, and find a restoration technique that worked for her. With a well-rounded daily program in place, Laura could improve her health both physically and mentally and not have to combat the side effects of multiple medications.

Initially daunted by the idea of changing her life so much, Laura was relieved to hear from Stephanie that she could make the changes gradually. Laura knew that the road she was headed down with the medications was not how she wanted to live her life. She was inspired to take better care of herself and had stopped taking all the medications by her next annual exam, at which she was radiant and excited to tell Stephanie the details of how she had turned her life around.

rating the techniques we suggest. In general, lower doses are associated with fewer side effects.

The use of medication for treatment of stress-related symptoms can be helpful but is complex and expensive. We believe you should try nonpharmaceutical options first.

The following chapter on nutrition will introduce you to the well-established therapeutic and nourishing benefits of food in keeping your body in balance.

# CHAPTER SIX

# NUTRITION

It is time to consider the nourishment your body needs to operate in top form. The essential purpose of the stress response is to provide you with a burst of energy either to escape a threat or to protect yourself by fighting, so, if you are stressed, you need the best fuel possible. In this chapter, we are not concerned with weight loss, although changing the way you eat as we advise might well have that effect. Instead, we want you to eat in a way that shows respect for the extraordinary gift of your body and that helps to keep all its systems functioning harmoniously and efficiently. Here we will provide you with the best ways to nourish your body to combat stress.

Food has three functions. The first is nutritional, which is essential to survival. The second is sensory, meaning that food satisfies sensory needs through a combination of flavor and texture. The third function is physiological: the foods you eat actually help regulate your biorhythms, the aging process, mood, and the immune system. Known as functional foods, these nutrients have health benefits that have been confirmed by medical research. We are particularly interested in functional foods in our approach to nutrition.

Good nutrition will make a significant contribution to rebalancing your damaging stress responses. If you are a HyperS, you can use food to calm you and support your suppressed immune function. You can eat foods that will give you optimal brain function and lower your tendency for insulin resistance by keeping your blood sugar steady. We will tell you which foods can help make your body less acidic and bring your cortisol levels down. If you are a HyperP, we will show you how to prevent your periodic crashes. Protein will help to replenish your neurotransmitter balance to restore you when you do crash. We'll tell you how to use food to increase your energy and support your immune system. If you identify with the HypoS type, you need to eat anti-inflammatory foods that counteract your aggressive immune system to prevent pain and fatigue. Timing your meals and balancing proteins and carbohydrates will help improve your cortisol production and entrain your desynchronized rhythm. If you're a HypoP, you will learn about foods that prevent abdominal cramping and intestinal disorders. You will also need to use food to stimulate cortisol production and to get your rhythm in sync.

Throughout this chapter there are general nutritional recommendations that apply to all four types and nutritional strategies that concern only one or two types. The appropriate icons appear at the beginning of each section. You'll want to jot down information that is pertinent to your type in your Stress Journal. The Stress-Detox Programs in chapter 9 will give you a personal prescription that tailors all the advice in this chapter into a strategic nutrition plan for your type.

## NATURAL TRANQUILIZERS

If you are not eating a healthful diet, you are stressing your body, whether or not you are under other emotional or environmental stress. Nutritional deficiency is a powerful stressor. A slight iron deficiency reduces the oxygen supply to your brain, which can make you irritable, tired, and unable to concentrate. If you are deficient in B vitamins, your cells' ability to convert carbohydrates and fats to energy is inhibited. A magnesium deficiency can make you sensitive to noise and crowds, escalating your stress levels.

When you are stressed, you are more vulnerable to nutritional deficiencies than ever, which means that your body's response to those deficiencies will increase your stress. If you are well nourished, you will be better able to cope with stress. The irony is that often our eating habits become totally disrupted under stress, when we need nutritional balance the most.

## A SIMPLE STRATEGY

Today, many people are eating food that is energy dense, meaning highly caloric, and nutritionally empty or even harmful because of additives, preservatives, and artificial sweeteners. With so much processed and prepackaged foods available for fast and tasty eating, it's easy to lose sight of the actual nutritional value of what you eat. Chemically enhanced flavors have become so prevalent that many people now prefer the intense sweetness of artificial flavors and have lost their appreciation for the subtle sweetness and varied textures of fresh, whole foods. Our philosophy of eating is simple: replace processed foods with fresh, whole, organic, local food as often as possible. We know it's easy for us to say, because we live in Southern California with its year-round growing season. But we guarantee that you will look better, feel better, and counteract the harmful impact of stress if you incorporate more healthy foods into your life.

Whole foods, in contrast to processed foods, are not adulterated in any way and contain all their original nutrients. Whole foods have the enzymes and other elements needed for your body to digest and assimilate what you have eaten. Whole foods are not refined or enriched and are nutritionally superior to highly refined processed foods—the foods you find in packages in the center aisles of a supermarket. A nutrient or chemical is added to food usually because natural nutrients were removed in processing. Your body has difficulty digesting and

### Real Life

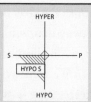

Sommer, thirty-one, complained to Stephanie about fatigue, headaches, and weight gain. She had a three-year-old son and a two-year-old daughter, who kept her busy. She seemed never to have a moment to herself. After examining her and talking with her for some time, Stephanie asked her what she had eaten the day before. Sommer thought about it a bit and smiled, confessing that she was embarrassed to say. She had grabbed a breakfast bar and washed it down with black coffee as she fed the children and had drunk a can of diet cola as she did household chores. For lunch, she had popped a frozen diet meal in the microwave. She'd had a large latte as she took the children for their annual check-up. Back at home, while they napped, she'd had a bag of chips along with more diet soda as she paid the bills at the computer. At the park that day, one of the mothers had baked some chocolate chip cookies she couldn't resist. Before her husband got home from work, she had fed the children and nibbled on leftover chicken tenders and some carrots. She'd thought she would make a simple pasta, salad, and garlic bread for dinner, but the greens had looked wilted and forlorn, so she'd decided to skip making a salad. Her husband had wanted pizza, so she'd had a pepperoni pie delivered with a salad—iceberg lettuce with a few carrot shavings. As they'd watched TV that night, she had a big bowl of ice cream.

Stephanie did not even have to comment. Sommer realized that she was eating badly. Stephanie recognized that Sommer was a mild HypoS stress responder. She advised Sommer to have fresh, wholesome food in the house for meals and snacks. After all, she made sure the children ate well; she owed herself the same consideration.

With a weekly plan in place, Sommer was able to prepare in advance for those busy days. She kept a day's supply of washed and cut vegetables—carrots, celery, bell peppers—in the refrigerator for snacking. She had cheese cut into squares for quick bites when she was hungry, kept nuts and berries handy for snacks, and carried bags of trail mix in her car. She planned simple, nutritious meals she could share with her children, such as roasted chicken, brown rice, broccoli, and a salad. She could even get two meals out of the chicken if she made a little extra and chicken tacos for lunch.

At her next visit with Stephanie, she was more energetic and said that her children were also healthier. They hadn't had a cold or sore throat in months. She felt the shift in their eating habits was well worth the effort.

using food when its composition is altered by preservatives, additives, dyes, microwaves, irradiation, and the manufacturer's cooking. If your diet relies heavily on processed foods, you are not nourishing your body adequately, and the stress of that poor nutrition will negatively affect your mind and spirit.

We're not going to present you with a food pyramid or tell you to have a certain number of portions of various foods a day. Each of the four types has different needs. What we will tell you is how to eat in a way that will protect your body from stress damage and keep your body in allostatic balance.

We want you to remember that a body starved for nutrients will keep eating until it obtains them. The more low-quality food you eat, the more you will want to eat. Since your diet might need improvement, we recommend that you keep a food log for a couple weeks. We provide you with a daily log at the end of "The Stress-Detox Programs," which you can follow in this book or copy into your Stress Journal. Many of our patients do keep a record and are frequently surprised to find that green vegetables rarely touch their lips or that diet cola and processed snack foods have become the main source of their energy. Recording what you eat in the course of a day and how you feel before and after you eat can be an eye-opening experience.

The benefits of eating whole grains are substantial. The fiber helps to lower cholesterol in the blood and puts the absorption of glucose on a time delay, so you don't get a sugar high or spike in your blood-sugar levels. Slower glucose absorption means that your body produces less insulin, also a good thing.

Fiber can prevent small blood clots by stimulating the body's natural anticoagulants. The vitamin E found in whole grains prevents LDL cholesterol from reacting with oxygen; over time, this reaction leads to clogged arteries. The layer of bran found in whole grains also supplies minerals, including magnesium, selenium, copper, and manganese, which can reduce the risk of developing heart disease. One study found that women who eat two and a half portions of whole grains a day are 30 percent less likely to develop heart disease than those who consume one serving a week.

It should not be difficult to incorporate more whole grains into your diet. Try substituting brown rice for white rice, whole-wheat pasta for white-flour pasta. You can also experiment with grains such as quinoa, amaranth, barley, buckwheat, bulgur, or whole-

> **Whole Food Nation**
>
> Paavo Airola, the nutritionist and naturopathic physician who was among the first
> health professionals to advocate the use of antioxidants against damage caused by
> free radicals, told a compelling story about the effects of healthful eating.
>     During World War I, Denmark suffered from grave food shortages. Dr. M. Hind-
> hede, who was the director of the Danish Institute of Nutrition Research at the time,
> was responsible for protecting the people from the threat of hunger. The government
> increased whole-grain production by limiting livestock and alcohol production,
> saving grain for human consumption. Farmers were directed to produce more grain,
> green vegetables, fruits, and dairy products. Grain processing was stopped to save
> energy, and only whole-grain products were sold. He reported that in one year, the
> death rate dropped 40 percent. According to Airola, Denmark became the healthiest
> country in Europe within a few years. The citizens of Denmark resisted the deadly
> influenza epidemic and other diseases that affected the rest of Europe at the time.
>     We are not expecting you to give up meat or the occasional martini, but this historic
> experiment dramatically shows the value of whole, unrefined foods.

wheat couscous. Try steel-cut oats for breakfast rather than instant oatmeal; steel-cut oats are digested more slowly than processed oatmeal and will leave you feeling fuller. Check labels with an eye for the word *whole*. Don't be fooled by labels that say "made with wheat flour." This does not mean that the product is made with whole wheat.

Stress depletes your body of nutrients, so it makes sense for you to eat foods that are as rich in nutrients as you can find and that will deliver nutrients in their most effective form. Organic food is grown and raised without poisons or hormones. We encourage you to eat organic foods rather than food that has been treated with chemicals that can interfere with your body's natural functioning. After all, you eat what your food eats. It's passed right on to you.

Food that is grown in a natural way rather than industrially has substantially more minerals, vitamins, and phytonutrients than commercially grown foods. Even more important, organic produce and meat are actually more flavorful and aromatic. Just compare the fla-

## Nutrition 101

**Macronutrients** are the principal constituents of food: carbohydrates, protein, fats, and water. **Carbohydrates,** which consist of sugar compounds, provide energy to the body. There are three types of carbohydrates:

- **Simple carbohydrates, or monosaccharides,** have one or two units of sugar. Examples are *fructose,* found in fruit, *glucose,* or blood sugar that is produced when carbohydrates are digested, and *galactose,* which is produced from digesting milk sugar, or lactose.

- **Disaccharides** are formed from two units of sugar; for example, table sugar, or *sucrose,* is composed of one unit of fructose and one of glucose.

- **Complex carbohydrates, or polysaccharides,** are formed by more than two units of sugar linking together. Thousands of simple sugars can be strung together in various structures, which is why there is such diversity in grains, fruits, and vegetables. Complex carbohydrates take two forms: starches and fiber. *Starches* can be digested, though cooking might be necessary, while digestive enzymes cannot break the bonds of the sugar units in *fibers,* including cellulose, pectin, beta-glucans, and gum.

- **Protein,** which means "of prime importance" in Greek, provides the body's essential building material. Protein is needed for the metabolic activity of every cell in your body. Enzymes, many hormones, neurotransmitters, and antibodies are made of protein. Each protein is a combination of amino acids. Body proteins are composed of twenty different amino acids. The body is capable of making eleven of these amino acids; the source of the other nine must come from your diet. There are a huge number of possible amino-acid combinations.

- **Fats (lipids)** provide another source of energy that is used in basal metabolism, stored for future use, supply fatty acids for chemical activities, carry the fat-soluble vitamins A, D, E, and K, and are at the root of flavor, texture, aroma, and fullness.

- **Simple lipids** are the most common fats in your body. They are burned for energy and are stored in the form of adipose tissue. The most familiar simple lipids are the triglycerides.

- **Essential fatty acids,** such as alpha-linolenic and linoleic acid, are not produced by the body but are supplied by what you eat. Omega-3 and omega-6 are important essential fatty acids. Essential fatty acids are saturated, unsaturated, and polyunsaturated. Each molecule of fatty acid is a chain of carbon atoms to which hydrogen atoms are bound. A fat is **saturated** if all the hydrogen atoms that could possibly bind are present. When hydrogen atoms are missing and two carbon atoms bind together, a bond is formed between the carbon atoms. Fatty acids with one such bond are **monounsaturated,** and—you guessed it—if two or more of these bonds exist, the fatty acid is **polyunsaturated.** Most fats are a combination of saturated, monounsaturated, and polyunsaturated molecules in varying proportions.

- **Trans fats** are man-made fats found in margarine, vegetable shortening, fast-food french fries, commercial baked goods, and processed foods. They raise LDL cholesterol and trigylcerides in your bloodstream, make blood platelets stickier, and contribute to inflammation.

- **Micronutrients** are vitamins and minerals.

- **Vitamins** are nutrients needed in small quantities that your body cannot make. They are either fat-soluble or water-soluble. **Fat-soluble** vitamins, such as vitamin A, can accumulate in the body, while **water-soluble** vitamins, such as vitamin C, do not. **Antioxidants,** such as vitamins C and E, stabilize free radicals, protecting cells and tissues by donating an electron to the volatile free radicals.

- **Minerals** are elements your body needs at trace levels for good health, including calcium, iron, magnesium, phosphorus, potassium, zinc, chlorine, copper, fluorine, manganese, selenium, sodium, and zinc.

vor of an organic turkey with a nonorganic one. The conventional, nonorganic turkey is so heavily treated that it can taste artificial and chemical, whereas the organic turkey has a much fresher, more distinct taste and texture. If you've never paid attention to what kind of produce you're buying, try it next time you go to the grocery store—you'll be amazed at the flavor difference and will probably start feeling better, too.

According to Michael Pollan in his extraordinary book *The Omnivore's Dilemma,* the entire food chain has been industrialized, degrading the chemical and biological qualities of our foods. Plants need nitrogen, phosphorus, and potassium in the soil to grow. Industrial fertilizer is synthesized from fossil fuels. Organic farming relies on the biological activity in the soil. Chemical fertilizers and pesticides reduce or destroy the complex underground ecosystem. Their use began in the 1950s, and the nutritional quality of our produce has declined ever since.

For example, plants produce polyphenols, which are potent antioxidants and are found in much higher levels in organic produce. Plants produce polyphenols to defend themselves against pests and disease, and the more exposure they have to these stressors, the more polyphenols they produce. When plants have the protection of pesticides, they no longer need to produce their own polyphenols to protect themselves, and the plant loses an important nutritional component. Plants grown in healthy soil that is rich in organic matter rather than chemicals produce more nutritious foods with higher levels of vitamins, minerals, antioxidants, and flavinoids (which give food flavor).

## SUPPORT YOUR LOCAL FARMER

When it comes to the benefit of buying local food, just consider the journey of a tomato you buy in the supermarket. The tomato is picked green so that it will not be bruised in shipping. It is sprayed with ethylene gas to turn it red. Since the tomato never really ripens, it tastes like pulp, with none of the delicious flavor of a fresh-picked tomato. Even organic produce that you buy in the supermarket has traveled a long way, possibly thousands of miles over days. The nutritional value of food deteriorates almost from the moment it's harvested, so freshly picked produce, even if it is not organic, trumps supermarket organic fruits and vegetables. Local produce will be tastier and be more nutritious. Also, small, local farmers often do not need pesticides, because they have a diversified crop.

# MICRONUTRITIONAL INSURANCE

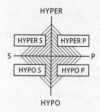

Although it is unquestionably better to deliver micronutrients in their natural state to your body, we recommend that you take a daily multivitamin. Few of us have a perfect diet, and it is impossible to measure your deficiencies and how stress is depleting your vitamins and minerals without medical tests. Of course, your needs vary from day to day, depending on what you eat, how you sleep, and how stressed you are. It makes sense to be certain that you are getting all the micronutrients you need by taking a multivitamin that includes minerals. But we do not want you to substitute taking supplements for eating well.

---

## Real Life

Kate had once been nearly one hundred pounds overweight. She was a HyperS responder with insulin resistance. She had struggled for three years to take off the weight; now that she had, she intended never to put it back on. She had lost the weight on a program that provided frozen, processed food, and she worried about portion control as she made the shift to real food. Kate was still in deprivation/diet mode: she used coffee to suppress her appetite, especially at lunch, and drank several cups every day. She was concerned when she came in for her yearly exam with Stephanie, because she didn't like her irritable moods, often felt edgy and anxious, and usually crashed in the late afternoon.

Stephanie advised Kate to wean herself gradually off the coffee over a period of a month to help prevent withdrawal symptoms. She recommended that Kate drink one or two cups of green tea daily to improve alertness and decrease her irritability. Stephanie also suggested that Kate needed to adjust her perspective about food: she had to consider food as nourishment for her body rather than as an enemy. After a long nutritional-counseling session about delicious, fresh, whole foods, Kate felt armed with useful information and began to make changes. She liked the idea that if she picked the right foods, she did not have to obsess about portion size. The next year, her weight was stable, and she was feeling as good as she looked.

Vitamins have been receiving a good deal of bad press lately. The Women's Health Initiative published a study in 2001 that examined the impact of hormone replacement therapy on heart disease, breast cancer, and colon cancer. An additional part of the study looked at multivitamin use by the nearly 165,000 women who participated. The results on multivitamin use were published in 2009. From their statistics on heart disease and colon cancer diagnosed during the study, they concluded that multivitamins were not effective in preventing cardiovascular disease and colon cancer in women age fifty and older. The media covered these findings with overstatements that did not provide the full story or context. Headlines announced VITAMIN PILLS: A FALSE HOPE? and STUDY FINDS NO BENEFIT FROM DAILY MULTIVITAMIN. This study was not designed primarily to examine the impact of multivitamins in preventing heart disease and colon cancer. Had this been the focus of the study, the process of data analysis and study design would have been different. For example, the multivitamins that the women took were not standardized. The participants were taking multivitamins with different content, doses, and quality. Finally, failure to show a direct link between taking multivitamins and the prevention of heart disease or colon cancer does not mean that taking vitamins does not have other benefits. We believe that taking a multivitamin can help to ensure that you are getting nutrients that might be missing from your diet or depleted by stress.

**The supplements we discuss in the list that follows are important for all stress types.** We will emphasize the importance of some for the individual types and will include the icons in the headings. You should of course consult your own physicians, but these are the basics we believe women need to ensure their micronutrient needs are covered.

### *Vitamin A*
### 700 IU to a maximum of 3000 IU

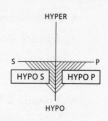

- Improves regeneration, adaptability, and production of brain cells, especially in the hippocampus, to help maintain memory and cognitive function under stress
- Helps to stabilize cellular membranes in the brain to ensure that neurons can function optimally
- Protects neural tissues from free-radical damage, also known as "oxidative stress"
- Vitamin A is more readily available and six times more powerful from animal than from vegetable sources, which puts vegetarians at risk for deficiency.
- People with inflammatory-bowel conditions are also at risk for vitamin A deficiency, because these conditions make it difficult to absorb fat-soluble vitamins, so this supplement is particularly important for the HypoS and the HypoP types.

Natural sources include liver, milk, butter, eggs, some cheeses, fish, green vegetables, carrots, yellow fruit, and oranges. (Vegetable oil increases the bioavailability of beta-carotene, a form of vitamin A.)

### *B Complex—Vitamins B1, 2, 3*
### 50 mg. to 100 mg.

- Vitamin B1 facilitates the brain's use of glucose for energy.
- Deficiency for just six days leads to impaired cognitive function, irritability, muscle cramps, and cardiac arrhythmias.
- Even a slight deficiency in B1 is associated with mood swings among women.

- B1 deficiency is more common in alcohol abusers.
- Animal studies have shown that B1 deficiency results in neuronal-cell death, particularly in the thalamus region of the brain.
- Vitamin B2, also known as riboflavin, is important to help balance the effects of B1 and B3. Deficiency is associated with migraines.
- Vitamin B3 is available in two forms, niacin and niacinamide. Since B3 has a calming effect on the brain, neurons can become overly excitable with a deficiency. It has been reported to reduce anxiety.
- B3 (niacin) can reduce cholesterol.
- At high doses of 1000 mg. daily, niacin can cause tingling or flushing that can feel like an allergic reaction. Niacinimide, the other form of B3, does not cause flushing but also does not lower cholesterol.

Natural sources include chicken, turkey, beef, fish, whole-grain bread, peanuts, lentils, lima beans, dairy products, and eggs.

### Vitamin B6 (pyridoxine)
**1.3 mg. to a maximum of 100 mg.**

- B6 is concentrated in the brain one hundred times more than in the blood.
- B6 helps convert stored carbohydrates and other nutrients to glucose to maintain energy supply to the brain when you are not eating enough.
- Needed for normal functioning of the more than one hundred enzymes used in protein metabolism
- Effective for relief of PMS and premenstrual depression

- Works with folic acid, vitamin B12, and tryptophan to produce serotonin
- Involved in the production of dopamine and GABA

Natural sources include potatoes, bananas, chickpeas, chicken, pork, beef, and fish. Women typically consume only half the recommended daily allowance of vitamin B6 in their diet. They consume less meat, a B6-rich food, than men do.

### *Vitamin B9—Folic Acid*
**400 micrograms to 1000 mg.**

HYPER

HYPER S | HYPER P

S ——————— P

HYPO

- Important for memory and intellectual capacity in elderly
- Important role in neuronal-cell growth and maintenance because it is involved in the production of DNA and RNA. Helps to protect the DNA from damage that can lead to cancer.
- Important in production of norepinephrine and serotonin. Necessary for HyperPs and HyperSs
- Important for fetal development during pregnancy. Supplementation helps prevent abnormal neurologic development that causes spina bifida. All pregnant women should take folic-acid supplements.

Natural sources: liver, eggs, watercress, spinach, leeks, lentils, asparagus, broccoli, cauliflower, corn, chickpeas, almonds, chestnuts, and black-eyed peas.

## Vitamin B12
### 5–12 micrograms a day

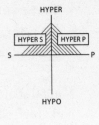

- Improves memory
- Deficiency results in neurological and psychiatric disturbances.
- Deficiency is associated with malaise or general feelings of illness.
- Plays a role in the production of energy from fats and proteins
- B12 is particularly important for HyperS and HyperP types because it is involved in the replenishment of norepinephrine levels.
- Vegetarians are at risk for severe deficiency, which can cause memory loss, pain, and abnormal sensations in the arms and legs.

Natural sources: foods of animal origin—meat, eggs, shellfish, fish, cheese, milk, and some algae.

## Vitamin C
### 75–3000 mg. per day

- Needed to transform dopamine to norepinephrine. Important for HyperSs and HyperPs for the same reasons as mentioned for vitamin B12.
- Has an anti-stress effect at high doses by reducing cortisol, blood pressure, and subjective responses to psychological stress. We recommend taking very high doses (1000 mg. three times per day) only in situations of acute stress.
- The adrenal and pituitary glands—the major stress glands—

are the primary storage sites for vitamin C. During stress, these stores are depleted, which can intensify the stress response.

- Has immune-boosting effects by increasing antimicrobial and natural killer-cell activities, and lymphocyte proliferation—another reason why it is important for the HyperS and HyperP types
- Has been shown to reduce irritability and fatigue
- Has an antioxidant effect

Natural sources include oranges, grapefruit, sweet red peppers, broccoli, tomatoes, strawberries, and potatoes.

### Vitamin D

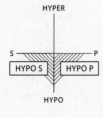

The dose of this supplement depends on your sun exposure. Blood tests are needed to determine dosage. If you use sunblock regularly, you may not be getting enough vitamin D. People with darker skin require longer sunlight exposure to make the same amount of vitamin D that fair-skinned people make.

- Synthesized in the skin from UVB radiation, or sunlight exposure
- When sunlight exposure is minimal, supplements should be taken.
- Vitamin D3 is the most bioavailable form.
- A blood test for vitamin level is important to determine the need for supplementation. The blood test should measure serum 25(OH)D levels.
- Time of day, season, and latitude influence our skin's production of vitamin D.

- Important for maintaining normal serum calcium concentrations, which affects bone density
- Involved in the stimulation of insulin production
- Shown to help prevent inflammatory bowel disease, which is particularly important for the HypoS and HypoP stress types.
- Modulates the activity of activated T and B lymphocytes, mitigating or preventing a wide variety of autoimmune disorders. Important for HypoS and HypoP types.
- Has mood-elevating effects
- Improves anxiety and depression

Food sources include salmon, mackerel, sardines, fortified milk, and eggs.

### *Vitamin E*
**15–1000 mg.**

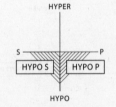

- A major antioxidant, providing protection from aging caused by free-radical damage especially in the brain
- Alpha-tocopherol is the most biologically active form and the only form that is recognized to meet human requirements. Check the label to make certain that alpha-tocopherol is the form of vitamin E you are buying.
- Helps prevent heart disease by aiding in the dilation of blood vessels and prevention of platelet aggregation
- Inflammatory-bowel issues make this fat-soluble vitamin difficult to absorb. Important for the HypoS and HypoP types who are prone to this type of problem

Natural sources include olive oil, canola oil, almonds, hazelnuts, peanuts, avocado, carrots.

### Zinc
**10–30 mg.**

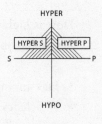

- Important for immune function. Even mild deficiency has been shown to impair the function of white blood cells.
- Important for DNA synthesis and cell division
- Required for a proper sense of taste and smell. This property particularly affects elderly people and can create a vicious cycle. As food becomes unappealing and an elderly person eats less as a result, the zinc deficiency can continue to worsen.
- Important for HyperS and HyperP to protect against immune-compromising effects of stress

Natural sources include oysters, shellfish, steak, chicken livers, yogurt, cashews, and cheese.

### Magnesium
**320 mg.**

- Helps maintain normal muscle and nerve function. Involved in the relaxation of muscles. Deficiency can be associated with muscle spasms and charley horses.
- Metabolism of carbohydrates, lipids, and proteins requires magnesium to produce the primary source of cellular energy, called ATP.
- Keeps the heart rhythm steady
- Promotes bone density

Natural sources include milk, water, snails, green beans, walnuts, sorrel, lentils, mussels, clams, spinach, beets, halibut, almonds, and soybeans.

*Calcium*
(Check with your doctor before starting calcium supplementation.) Most common mineral in the human body and the major structural element of bones and teeth, calcium is needed to prevent osteoporosis.

- Plays a role in the constriction and dilation of blood vessels
- Involved in the conduction of nerve impulses, muscle constriction, and insulin secretion
- Has been shown to improve PMS possibly through serotonin production, but the exact mechanism is unknown.

Natural sources include dairy products, pinto beans, red beans, white beans, tofu, bok choy, spinach, broccoli, kale, cabbage, and rhubarb.

*Iron*
Dose is highly dependent on need, so blood tests are needed to determine dose.

- Has an important role in oxygen transport and storage
- Deficiency eventually leads to anemia, impaired production of the oxygen-carrying molecule, or hemoglobin, in the blood.
- Even before anemia develops, deficiency can lead to symptoms such as apathy, sleepiness, irritability, inability to concentrate, and memory loss.
- Low levels lead to a lower supply of oxygen to the brain.
- Low levels can reduce the brain's energy production by decreasing activity of cytochrome c oxidase, an important enzyme in certain brain regions.
- Deficiency during pregnancy can cause long-term cognitive deficits in children.

- Dietary iron is more bioavailable in the form of heme iron, found mostly from animal sources.
- Dietary iron from plant sources is highly dependent on what you eat with your vegetables. Tea will decrease the absorption and orange juice will enhance it. Meat increases the absorption of iron found in vegetables. Soybeans slightly decrease the absorption.

Natural sources include beef, poultry, shellfish, fish, molasses, raisins, prunes, potatoes, kidney beans, lentils, tofu, and cashews.

## SUPPLEMENT QUALITY

There is great variability in the quality of dietary supplements. Though some companies do research, manufacture, and sell their own supplements, most dietary supplements are produced by a few dozen companies and repackaged by other companies with their own labels. Supplements do not have to be expensive to be of high quality. The box on page 142 will give you some ways to evaluate the quality of supplements.

## HOW YOUR BODY KNOWS WHAT AND WHEN TO EAT

Since we need food to survive, our bodies have an intricate system in place to ensure that we nourish them properly. A gut–brain axis exists that controls appetite and meal size. These nutrient-sensing pathways are an allostatic system that regulates energy balance. The system is affected by many factors, including genetics, circadian rhythm, reproductive cycle, and age. When you perceive hunger, neural mechanisms have stimulated your appetite. As you eat, your digestive system sends signals about the quantity and the quality of food you have consumed to your

**Quality Control**

You can learn about the quality of dietary supplements by checking the labels and packaging. Dietary supplements are not regulated, so the content of the pills might differ from what is listed on the label. Jeffrey Moss, DDS, CNS, DACBN, of Moss Nutrition, helped to clarify some terms that are marketing tools. The word *natural* is meaningless on a label, because every supplement is derived from processed food; its natural state is the actual food it's derived from. Do some research online before you invest in supplements.

- Look for the ConsumerLab.com quality seal on the label or package or join Consumerlab.com to find out which brands they have tested. The company has an independent testing program and the products that they endorse are of high quality.

- The USP or NF seal indicates that the producer claims that the supplement meets the U.S. Pharmacopoeia or National Formulary standards for that product. These standards cover minimum dosage, potency, and purity.

- The National Nutritious Foods Association (NNFA) awards a GMP (Good Manufacturing Practice) seal that indicates the manufacturer has passed a comprehensive inspection of its manufacturing process. Though the seal assures that the supplement is well made, it does not judge the manufacturer's ingredients and potency levels.

- The BioFit trademark means that the product has passed biological assay testing, meaning that its biochemical activity during the test has a corresponding effect in the human body.

- SupplementWatch.com uses a one-hundred-point rating system for brands. Up to twenty points are awarded for each of five categories: health claims, scientific theory, scientific research, safety and side effects, and value.

- If none of this gives you the information you need, ask the lab that made the vitamins how they test their products. Most reputable companies will have professionals who can answer your questions. According to Jeffrey Moss, you will want to ask them about toxicology and microbiology reports as well as a postproduction analysis.

- Look for an expiration date to be certain that the product is fresh. If there is no expiration date on the label, do not buy the supplement.

brain. Your body communicates with your brain about the availability of fuels for the long and the short term. The micronutrients in your meal can have significant effects on your nervous system, particularly the structure and function of the neurons. Macronutrients in the foods you eat provide energy for your body and brain.

## FOOD AND THE CIRCADIAN RHYTHM

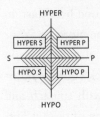

As we have discussed, the level of cortisol in your body rises and falls on a twenty-four-hour rhythm, with highest concentrations just as you are about to wake up in the morning and lowest at around midnight. When you eat is an important synchronizer and organizer of the circadian rhythm of cortisol secretion. As we have mentioned, this is extremely important for the HypoS and HypoP stress types, whose cortisol levels are low or desynchronized.

In anticipation of your usual mealtime, your body prepares to use the energy you are about to consume. Norepinephrine and cortisol levels rise and fall in a specific pattern at mealtimes that coordinate the pathways of energy storage and utilization. Eating provides a link between the hormonal pathways and metabolism.

Skipping breakfast is a bad idea. Your circadian rhythm has signaled your body that the day has begun, and cortisol and the natural rhythms of your body have prepared you to receive and use nutrients efficiently at this time. Lunch is associated with a midday peak in cortisol. A lunch that is too large can make you sluggish and lethargic, because it will raise your insulin levels. Afternoon snacks can help cognitive performance, and going from lunch to dinner without an energy boost can be stressful to your body. We recommend that in order to steady your blood-sugar levels, you should have a small snack of nuts, fruit, or yogurt at three or four o'clock in the afternoon. Studies have shown dinner can energize you for one to three hours after you eat, as the evening meal causes a rise in cortisol. If you eat too close to bedtime, this rise in cortisol may interfere with your circadian rhythm and disrupt your sleep.

Whatever your type, you have to consider potential circadian-rhythm problems. Since HyperSs and HyperPs have an entrained cortisol rhythm, your meal timing is not as important as it is for the other two types. Since both Hyper types tend to have nervous stomachs, you should eat small meals throughout the day. Have a good breakfast, in particular, because you are less insulin-resistant in the morning. Your insulin production lags behind your morning cortisol pulse, so you can eat more at breakfast without gaining weight. Pack your breakfast with nutrient-dense foods such as eggs scrambled with spinach and tomatoes or other seasonal vegetables or a tablespoon of peanut butter on whole-grain toast. Some protein is important. Have a slice of grapefruit with these other foods, as it will help neutralize the pH (balance the acid and alkaline foods) of your breakfast (we will explain more about pH later). Have some berries and yogurt. **Hyper stress responders should not drink coffee until after breakfast.** If you must drink it, wait an hour or two until after breakfast, because it will interfere with the absorption of the nutrition you are getting. Try green tea instead of coffee. It has less caffeine but is still stimulating and has the additional health benefits of a rich supply of antioxidants. It won't interfere with the absorption of your morning nutrients.

If you're HypoS or HypoP, you need to use food to stimulate the rhythmic production of cortisol and to balance your overly active sympathetic nervous system, which will lessen your pains and fatigue. Studies of cortisol levels in human saliva have shown that high-protein lunches compared with high-protein meals at other times of the day or with meals high in carbohydrates are associated with the biggest release of cortisol. A large lunch high in protein should be your goal. A Cobb salad is an excellent choice. You need to remember to be very

**Real Life**

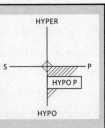

Erin is a young mother of two. Her four-month-old still awakens several times a night. She is up with him every time he wakes up to nurse him and finds it difficult to fall back asleep. Since the children rarely nap at the same time, Erin doesn't get to catch up on sleep. Her schedule is erratic. Sometimes she gets up at 5:00 a.m., after the baby has awakened her; at other times, she sleeps until 7:00 a.m. She goes to bed early on some nights and late on others. Beth asked about her nutrition and her eating schedule, but Erin drew a blank; during this postpartum period her focus was completely on the children. Erin related her story to Beth with little expression or emotion. When questioned, she told Beth that she did not usually spend time with friends, but occasionally with family. She was shy and withdrawn, a HypoP stress responder. Beth believed that Erin's circadian rhythm would have needed entrainment even if she were not dealing with young children and suggested that Erin might benefit from psychological therapy. She suggested that Erin begin to put herself on a schedule that coordinated with one for the children. Erin had to develop a routine, eating at a specific time in the morning, at lunch, and at dinner. Beth recommended that Erin take morning walks with the kids in a stroller outdoors to improve her mood. At a follow-up visit, having followed Beth's advice, Erin looked brighter and felt more energetic.

specific and consistent in the timing of your meals, as this will help synchronize your body's rhythms. Eat three meals per day at traditional times. The specific hour is not as important as consistency on a daily basis.

## THE WAGES OF STRESS

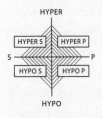

Stress is likely to disrupt your eating habits and, depending on your stress type, it might affect your eating habits in different ways. You might skip meals if you are a HyperS or a HyperP, because your appetite tends to be suppressed. You also are more likely to struggle with addictions to things like coffee, alcohol, and cigarettes, which you likely turn to in order to help you calm down. Your eating is suppressed due to the appetite-suppressing effects of CRH that is released at the start of the stress response. As you recover from stress, one of the lingering effects of cortisol is to stimulate your appetite for comfort foods and sweets. Eating habitually in this way can lead to allostatic load. Pay attention to your tendencies and make sure you eat three nutritious meals a day and have small, healthy snacks so that your body can obtain the nutrients and energy it needs to deal with your highly aroused state. A diet high in fat will keep your cortisol levels elevated, which limits your body's attempt to restore balance. We suggest you replace sweets and artificially sweetened desserts and snacks with fresh fruits. Limit your alcohol consumption to three to five drinks a week. Though a drink can be relaxing, more than that number will interfere with your sleep and will contribute to allostatic load.

If you are a HypoS and a HypoP, your stress sensitivity leads you to seek comfort from food. Comforting foods can stimulate endorphin production, especially foods that are both sugary and creamy. Endorphins are natural pain relievers, and, since you are highly prone to chronic pain, you may turn to comfort foods in an unconscious effort to deal with your pain. When you have a craving, we suggest you eat a piece of dark chocolate. The chocolate will calm the craving and boost your endorphin production. Dark chocolate is less processed and has less sugar than other types of chocolate. Snacks high in fiber are another good choice for you and will make you feel satisfied. Your digestion will benefit. You are prone to irritable-bowel function, especially under stress, so the increase in fiber will help you with this problem.

Since stress increases the breakdown of glycogen to glucose, slows down your digestion, and shunts blood from your stomach to your muscles, your body is not able to absorb nutrients as efficiently as it normally can. Your daily requirements will change and increase, because stress depletes your body of vitamins and minerals. Chronic stress depletes stores of vitamin C, an important antioxidant. The adrenal glands and pituitary gland are key storage sites for vitamin C, and when these glands are engaged in the HPA-axis response to stress, the stores of this important antioxidant are depleted. To intensify the problem, a diet that is high in calories but low in nutrients, typical of stress eating, depletes the B vitamins. A diet high in sugar can increase the urinary loss of magnesium and chromium, which are calming minerals.

## DIETS MAKE YOU EAT MORE WHEN STRESSED

Studies have found that men and women who diet regularly are more inclined to overeat. Women and restrained eaters or dieters consume more calories and fat under stress and turn to snack foods rather than

### Real Life

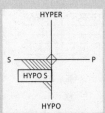

Sonja was a hardworking marketing executive. At her annual exam, she complained of weight gain and anxiety. Her job had been busy as usual, but her husband had fractured his leg while skiing and needed surgery. He would have a long recuperation during which he was completely incapacitated.

She loved caring for him in some ways, but he was in a lot of pain and could be irritable and demanding. She knew how frustrating being inactive was for him, but she found the situation overwhelming at times.

In the evenings after dinner, she craved sweets or chips and dip. She would sit in front of the TV while her husband was sleeping and mindlessly devour a huge bowl of ice cream or whole bags of chips. Her weight was going up, which was distressing to her.

Sonja had HypoS tendencies, so her body was seeking carbohydrates and fats to soothe her mind. Beth recommended that Sonja eat more foods containing tryptophan, such as eggs, chicken, and fish, and to combine these high-quality proteins with complex carbohydrates such as whole-grain pasta and vegetables at dinner. Beth suggested that Sonja enjoy a small piece of dark chocolate, which has soothing properties, and recommended that Sonja not eat once the TV was turned on. That way she could enjoy what she ate without distraction and stop adding the mindless calories in the evening.

nutritious foods. Men and women who do not diet showed little difference or a reduction in the foods they ate under stress.

Many popular diets achieve weight loss by denying the body specific nutrients: some are designed to lower your fat intake, others your carbohydrates. When you restrict your food intake to a very specific list of dos and don'ts, you are likely depriving your body of important macro- and micronutrients. If your brain is not receiving what it knows you need, you will find yourself looking to eat more. This is why most people gain weight back after they have been dieting for a while—the brain continues to look for what it needs to achieve allostatic balance.

## THINK BEFORE YOU DRINK

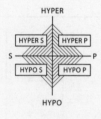

Beverages are a major source of calories in our diets but not always a good source of energy or nutrition. Between 1977 and 1996, the proportion of our energy that came from consuming caloric sweeteners rose 22 percent. The largest source of the added sugars comes from nondiet soft drinks. Americans increased their consumption of soda by 135 percent between 1977 and 2001. One twelve-ounce can of soda provides forty to fifty grams of sugar in the form of high-fructose corn syrup, the equivalent of ten teaspoons of sugar. In addition to carbonated soda, high-fructose corn syrup is found in sugar-sweetened iced tea, fruit drinks, many flavored waters, and sports drinks.

A number of studies have shown that sugar-sweetened drinks can lead to obesity and weight gain, because calories you drink are less satisfying than those derived from solid food, compelling you to eat more at your next meal. Others have found that when people increase their caloric intake by drinking sugar-sweetened beverages, they do not appropriately reduce the amount of solid food they eat. High-

## Sugar Substitutes Are Not the Answer

Our bodies judge how many calories a food contains by how it tastes. Sugar substitutes such as saccharin, sucratose, and neotame separate the taste of sweetness from the calories. The taste buds communicate to the brain that energy is coming in, but the body does not get the fuel it expects. Artificial sweeteners can interfere with your body's natural regulating processes and can upset your food chemistry. In a human study, those who ate aspartame-sweetened chocolate had higher rises in endorphins than did people who ate chocolate sweetened with sugar. Since artificial sweeteners are two hundred to thirteen thousand times as sweet as sugar, they can trick the body. The elevation in endorphins in response to an extremely sweet signal translates to increased pleasure, which could lead to eating more. The taste of sweetness is mildly addictive. The more sweets you eat, the more you need to feel satisfied.

fructose corn syrup may lead to greater weight gain and insulin resistance, because it decreases the production of insulin and leptin and does not suppress ghrelin, which means that the central nervous system does not receive fullness signals and continues to stimulate your appetite pathways. When you drink sweetened beverages, you are consuming more calories than your brain registers.

If you are a HyperS, HyperP, or HypoS, you are susceptible to insulin resistance, and this caution about sweetened beverages is particularly important for you. Insulin resistance is not the only problem with sweetened beverages. They also promote inflammation. This is another reason why HypoSs should avoid these drinks.

All stress types need to pay attention to their daily intake of water. Water is our most important nutrient after oxygen, essential to our health and emotional well-being. Sixty-five to 75 percent of an adult's body is composed of water, and a baby's is 90 percent. Water forms a large part of the foods we consume, particularly fruits and vegetables. Fruits, at 85 percent, have the highest level of water, and vegetables have slightly less. Cooked grains are 70 percent water.

Water is necessary for all body processes as it helps to regulate the temperature of the body; surrounds, fills, and nourishes cells and

**Cautionary Note on Caffeine**

Just one cup of coffee or a can of cola can directly affect your central nervous system. Caffeine affects your thought processes and coordination and increases your heart rate and respiration. Even more important, caffeine consumed with food can significantly reduce mineral absorption, particularly iron. It also drains your body of calcium and magnesium. The effects can last for hours.

We recommend that HyperS types avoid caffeine, because they need no additional stimulation. The other stress types should drink caffeine only occasionally and in moderation. Taper off gradually. Reducing your intake by four to six ounces every three days should keep you from having headaches, moodiness, and sluggishness. You might want to replace coffee or colas with chamomile, peppermint, or green tea, or just a couple of slices of fresh lemon in hot water instead.

tissues; transports nutrients, including oxygen, throughout your body; and helps to rid the body of toxins. Water is important in maintaining a healthy pH balance, which stabilizes nerves and tissues. Water washes out the various waste products that result from the normal function of your body. An accumulation of these compounds can cause you to feel tired; chronic low-grade dehydration is very common and is one of the causes of fatigue. Your body can mistake thirst for hunger. **If you crave a big bowl of ice cream, drink one or two glasses of water first. Water will curb your appetite and might stop those late-night munchies.**

Though the standard recommendation is to drink six to eight glasses of water a day, that may be excessive. A diet of two thousand calories a day requires sixty-four ounces of fluid, but that sixty-four ounces includes any beverage you drink as well as the water present in your food. The more fruits and vegetables you eat, the less water your body will need, whereas a diet heavy on meat, eggs, or salt will require more water. If you are physically active and work out a lot, you will need more water than will a woman who is sedentary. If you live in a hot, dry, windy climate, your water requirements will be high. To get the full benefits of hydration, try to avoid quenching your thirst with beverages that contain sugar or caffeine. If you are optimally hy-

**From the Bench**

A study from the University of Alberta found that women who experience PMS drink significantly less water than other women do. Perhaps these women were concerned that drinking too much water would increase fluid retention, but not drinking enough water actually causes your body to retain fluids. In fact, reducing salt intake and consuming more water helps the body to excrete excess fluid. A complex process, PMS makes us more vulnerable to stress, because our hormone fluctuations affect our major neurotransmitter systems and make us more susceptible to irritability and mood changes. By remaining adequately hydrated during this time, you can alleviate some of the symptoms of PMS, including bloating, swelling, and breast tenderness.

drated, your urine during the day should look clear and light (but not necessarily first thing in the morning).

## BE SURE TO STAY HYDRATED WHEN YOU EXERCISE

Since exercise makes you perspire, you have to replace that water loss. If you are outside and plan to exercise for more than thirty minutes, take water with you. Drink before you work out, every twenty minutes while you work out, and after you have finished to ensure that you remain adequately hydrated. But remember, drinking a beverage other than water could undo some of the great effects that exercise has. In particular, steer clear of the popular energy drinks that contain caffeine, high-fructose corn syrup, or artificial sweeteners. They may give you an immediate boost, but their effects are contrary to your exercise and stress-reducing goals.

## pH, ANOTHER BALANCING ACT

Fluids comprise 70 percent of our body weight, the same percentage of water to land on earth. The fluids in your body are acid, neutral, or alkaline. In order for all the systems in your body to function at optimal levels, the systems need the sea inside to border on being alkaline. This range is measured by pH on a scale of zero to fourteen.

The higher your pH is, the more alkaline the balance in your internal fluid will be; the lower your pH, the more acidic. For homeostasis, your blood pH should be 7.4, just slightly alkaline, and the average urine pH should be between 6.8 to 7.2, close to neutral. Cells function at their peak when pH is slightly alkaline. Purified water has a neutral pH balance of 7.0.

Paying attention to the pH of your foods is especially important for all four stress types. Acidic pH is associated with physical stress. If you are a HyperS or HyperP and your diet is too acidic, your excessive cortisol production will be compounded by an acidic pH. HypoS and HypoP types need proper pH to balance and counter the effects of inflammation.

pH controls intracellular activity, regulates your digestive system, and determines how your body uses enzymes, minerals, and vitamins. The normal pH for all tissues and fluids is alkaline, except for the stomach, which produces acidic enzymes for digestion. When your body converts food to energy, the processes of digestion and assimilation create by-products that can be acidic. The components of the modern Western diet—coffee, processed foods, dairy, and a lack of fresh produce—promote excess acidity. If acid levels in your body become too high, your body is unable to excrete the acid efficiently to return to balance. An acidic internal environment leads to degeneration and disease.

Stress can make your body acidic, which is the most common pH imbalance today. When all systems are functioning normally, there are adequate intracellular reserves of calcium and other minerals to meet the emergency demands required by the stress response. When your body's pH balance is overly acidic, the calcium and minerals that are used for normal function of your cells, especially in your bones, leave the cells and enter the bloodstream to alkalinize the pH. These cells become depleted of these minerals. If excessive acid is not neutralized, the alkaline reserves in your body will eventually be depleted in the attempt to do so. Bringing your pH into balance is an essential part of our Stress-Detox Programs. What you eat can make your body more, or less, acidic.

## CONDITIONS ASSOCIATED WITH LONG-TERM ACIDIC pH

Acidosis, an increase of acidity in the blood and extracellular fluid, can weaken every system in your body and leech minerals from your bones and organs. Some of the symptoms and diseases related to acidosis are:

- Weight gain
- Loss of skin elasticity (wrinkles)
- Joint pain
- Aching muscles
- Constipation
- Urinary-tract problems
- Stomachaches
- Nausea
- Kidney stones
- Chronic fatigue
- Loss of vitality
- Immune deficiency
- Gastritis
- Ulcers
- Obesity
- Diabetes
- Osteopenia and osteoporosis
- Gout
- Constriction of blood vessels
- Circulatory and cardiovascular weakness

Notice that these diseases can affect all stress types. pH issues are important for all.

There is a limit to what your body can do to reverse acid/alkaline imbalance, but there is something you can do from the outside: a sig-

**Looks Can Fool You**

It might not seem to make sense to incorporate more lemon into your diet, because it seems so acidic, but lemons have a high concentration of alkaline minerals. The acids in lemons are mild, organic ones that actually act as cleansing agents in your stomach.

nificant way to balance your pH is through your diet. Food shapes the pH environment in which your cells live. Good nutrition helps to build slightly alkaline extracellular fluid so that the cells can absorb nutrients, discharge toxins, and function at optimal levels that promote the proper function of your kidneys, liver, large intestine, and skin. The only way to build your body's reserves of the buffering minerals—calcium, sodium, potassium, and magnesium—is to eat an alkalizing diet with mineral and vitamin supplements. The key to alkalizing nutrition is to eat enzyme-rich fresh fruits and vegetables. The ideal balance is 80 percent alkaline-forming foods and 20 percent acid-forming foods.

To alkalinize your diet, consider making these changes:

- Eat less meat
- Decrease the amount of fat you consume
- Eat fewer pasteurized dairy products
- Avoid white sugar
- Eat more fruits and vegetables, especially raw for maximum nutrition
- Eat more nuts, seeds, and whole grains
- Use fresh lemon

## Acid- and Alkaline-forming Foods

| Most acidic | Acidic | Low acid | Low alkaline | Alkaline | Most Alkaline |
|---|---|---|---|---|---|
| NutraSweet Equal Aspartame Sweet'N Low | White sugar Brown sugar | Processed honey Molasses | Raw honey Raw sugar | Maple syrup | Stevia |
| Blueberries Cranberries Prunes | Sour cherries Rhubarb Unripe fruit | Plums Processed fruit juices | Oranges Bananas Cherries Pineapple Peaches Avocados | Dates Figs Melons Kiwi Berries Apples Pears Raisins | Lemons Watermelon Limes Grapefruit Mangoes Papayas |
| Sauerkraut | Skinless potatoes Pinto beans Navy beans Lima beans | Cooked spinach Kidney beans String beans | Carrots Tomatoes Fresh corn Mushrooms Cabbage Peas Potato skins Olives Soybeans Tofu | Okra Squash Green beans Beets Celery Lettuce Zucchini Sweet potato Carob | Asparagus Onion Vegetable juices (fresh) Parsley Leaf spinach Broccoli |
| Peanuts Walnuts | Pecans Cashews | Pumpkin seeds Sunflower seeds | Chestnuts | Almonds | |
| Processed oils | | Corn oil | Canola oil | Flaxseed oil | Olive oil Raw apple-cider vinegar |
| Wheat White flour Pastries Pasta | White rice Corn Buckwheat Oats Rye | Sprouted wheat Bread Spelt Brown rice | Amaranth Millet Wild rice | | |

| Most acidic | Acidic | Low acid | Low alkaline | Alkaline | Most Alkaline |
|---|---|---|---|---|---|
| Beef<br>Pork<br>Shellfish | Turkey<br>Chicken<br>Lamb | Venison<br>Cold-water fish | | | |
| Cheese<br>Pasteurized<br>  milk<br>Ice cream<br>Chocolate | Eggs<br>Butter<br>Yogurt<br>Buttermilk<br>Cottage cheese | Raw milk<br>Whey | Soy cheese<br>Soy milk<br>Goat milk<br>Goat cheese | | |
| Beer<br>Soft drinks | Coffee<br>Alcohol | Tea | Ginger tea | Green tea | Herb teas<br>Lemon and hot<br>water |

The signs and symptoms of pH imbalance can be subtle and non-specific. You may feel fatigued and lethargic, symptoms that are associated with many other imbalances as well. This imbalance is not an immediate health risk, but paying attention to the pH of your foods will aid in the prevention of chronic disease. You can test your pH easily at home with pH tester strips from your local drugstore.

## THE HUNGRY BRAIN

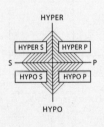

It takes a lot of energy to be conscious and to run your body; your brain consumes 20 percent of the energy generated by your body, even though it comprises only 2 percent of your body weight. At rest, your brain uses more than 50 percent of your dietary carbohydrates and consumes energy at ten times the rate of the rest of your body per gram of tissue.

Your brain needs nutrients to build and maintain its structure, to function smoothly, and to increase longevity. A deficiency in your diet can alter your cognitive skills and mood. Different cells require spe-

## From the Bench

### HIGH TEA

Tea, a rich source of flavonoid antioxidants, is the most widely consumed beverage in the world. Tea leaves contain L-theanine, an amino acid rarely found in nature, which appears to affect brain function in humans. A number of EEG studies of the human brain have shown that L-theanine relaxes the mind without inducing drowsiness. Additional studies have found that L-theanine is most effective with anxious people.

A team of researchers from the Netherlands and Oxford University has found that dietary levels of L-theanine have a significant effect on mental alertness and attention. L-theanine crosses the blood-brain barrier and takes effect within thirty minutes. Their conclusion was that L-theanine has a role in achieving a relaxed but alert mental state by directly influencing the central nervous system and increasing the alpha attention effect. So, if you are flagging, brew some tea rather than a pot of coffee. For these specific benefits, we are referring to tea made from real tea leaves and not herbal teas, though herbals can have their own set of benefits.

cific nutrients to play their part in your brain functions. The macronutrients, micronutrients, eight essential amino acids, and two essential fatty acids are all needed to maintain equilibrium.

## MACRONUTRIENTS, TRYPTOPHAN, AND TYROSINE, AND YOUR BRAIN

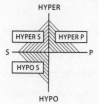

Tryptophan, an amino acid, is a precursor of serotonin. Tryptophan—along with vitamins B6, B12, and folic acid—is needed to produce serotonin, the neurotransmitter that calms you, improves your sleep, boosts your mood, decreases irritability, curbs your carbohydrate cravings, and increases your tolerance to pain.

The tryptophan needed to produce serotonin must be provided by what you eat, namely high-quality proteins. If you are a HyperS or a HypoS, you need typtophan in your diet to calm your highly revved central nervous system. HypoS types also need tryptophan to increase tolerance to pain, improve mood, and moderate the tendency to react intensely to stress.

**Sources of tryptophan include chicken, turkey, beef, lamb, fish, milk, yogurt, cheese, eggs, soybeans, almonds, cashews, peanuts, and sunflower seeds.**

Tryptophan competes with other amino acids you have eaten to cross the blood-brain barrier. After you eat carbohydrates, the pancreas produces more insulin, which causes the competing amino acids to leave the bloodstream and enter muscle tissues. With the other amino acids otherwise engaged, tryptophan can cross the blood-brain barrier, resulting in drowsiness. As you age, the amount of tryptophan that crosses the blood-brain barrier decreases.

A protein-rich meal without carbohydrates lowers brain tryptophan. You need carbohydrates as well as protein to produce serotonin. That is why a carbohydrate-rich snack can boost your mood. Another minus for caffeine is that it decreases the conversion of tryptophan to serotonin, one of the reasons why coffee can make you jittery. Increasing your brain serotonin may improve your ability to cope with stress, while a decline can lead to a depressed mood.

Tyrosine, another amino acid, shares entry into the brain with tryptophan through the same process. Tyrosine is involved with norepinephrine, epinephrine, and dopamine. Dopamine and norepiniphrine make you alert, vigilant, and better able to concentrate under stress and normal conditions.

If you are a HyperP type, be sure to get plenty of tyrosine in your diet. Getting enough tyrosine will help you prevent your crash days, which result because you really need more tyrosine. Include sources of tyrosine and complex carbohydrates at every meal, as this will restore your depleted norepinephrine levels more quickly.

**Sources of tyrosine include beef, chicken liver, game meats, fish, avocados, bananas, tofu, soybeans, red plums, raisins, sauerkraut, spinach, tomatoes, carrots, chickpeas, potatoes, brown rice, oats, nuts**

(especially almonds), beer, red wine, port, vermouth, and distilled spirits.

---

### Real Life

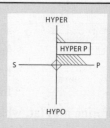

Anna is a busy working mother who teaches school so that she can be free to be with her three children after they have finished school. She loves being able to take them to all their after-school activities, but complained to Beth that she lacked energy on the weekends, was anxious and tired, and, on some Saturdays, just couldn't focus, exercise, or function as she usually did.

Beth found out that her nutrition was off. On a normal day, she told Beth, she grabs a granola bar and a yogurt on her way out the door and eats them as she waits for the school bus to pick up her children before she drives to the school at which she teaches. She buys a sandwich for lunch at the school cafeteria and wolfs it down with one eye on the students. Then she picks at the food as she prepares dinner. The children eat before their father arrives home from work. She usually does not sit down to eat with her husband, because she is helping her kids with their mountains of homework.

Beth explained the HyperP stress response to Anna and told her that the quality of the foods she was eating sounded reasonable, although she could use more fruits and vegetables. Anna also needed time to appreciate the foods she was eating and to slow down at mealtimes. Instead of a granola bar, Beth suggested that Anna eat a bowl of organic granola in the morning and that she savor every crunchy bite. Beth recommended that Anna take her lunch to school—a salad, cut-up vegetables with yogurt, leftovers from dinner the night before. She explained to Anna that she needed to incorporate tyrosine into her diet and gave her a list of tyrosine-rich foods.

She asked Anna to consider turning dinner into family time, when everyone could talk about what had happened that day and enjoy one another and the food she had prepared. It all made sense to Anna, who really did want to slow down to enjoy her life and her family more.

## STAYING ON AN EVEN KEEL

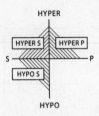

The demand for energy in your body is constant, and your brain in particular needs a steady, even supply of glucose to function at its best. The glucose level in your bloodstream is regulated by another hormonal balancing act, the insulin/glucagon axis. Insulin is responsible for taking excess energy and storing it as fat, while glucogen mobilizes energy. Insulin acts to drive down blood-sugar levels by stimulating cells to absorb the glucose carried in the bloodstream and to store it as fat. If your blood-glucose levels go below a critical level, your brain will signal for more glucose. A vicious cycle begins that will lead to more and more weight gain.

If glucose is not delivered to your hungry brain, your mind tunes out and you experience mental fatigue and a dramatic mood change, called "hypoglycemia," or low blood sugar. Hypoglycemia can lead to fatigue, irritability, palpitations, headaches, anxiety, difficulty concentrating, paleness, and shakiness. One way to counter this condition is to eat several small meals to keep blood sugar stable. The meals should consist of fiber-rich carbohydrates and protein.

HyperSs, HypoSs, and HyperPs are susceptible to blood-sugar swings and insulin resistance. Both excess cortisol and an overstimulated sympathetic nervous system can provoke insulin resistance. If you are one of these types, you need to understand how to keep your blood sugar steady and minimize the impact of insulin resistance on your health. Insulin resistance from a chronically activated fight-or-flight response is responsible for much of the allostatic load that develops with the HyperS type. HypoSs need to pay close attention to the following pages, as their tendency for insulin resistance along with low cortisol makes it difficult for them to recover from blood-sugar levels that fall too quickly.

Insulin resistance results when your cells, especially your muscle cells, no longer respond to insulin. Blood sugar stays at high levels, which forces the pancreas to produce more insulin in an effort to control your high-blood-sugar levels. If this state persists, the insulin-producing cells can wear out, resulting in type 2 diabetes. With diabetes, the body either does not release adequate insulin or does not use it efficiently, resulting in chronically elevated blood sugar. Several factors, other than chronic stress, influence the likelihood of your developing insulin resistance: obesity, inactivity, the dietary fats you consume, and genetics. Current research has also found a link between insulin resistance and breast cancer, colon cancer, and polycystic ovary syndrome.

An effective way to manage your blood sugar is with your diet. The insulin/glucogon balance is based on the size of a meal and its ratio of carbohydrates to protein. Insulin production is stimulated by eating carbohydrates and glucagon is stimulated by protein. What you eat can help to maintain the right hormonal balance to keep your blood sugar at optimal levels. When you eat carbohydrates, your

### Glycemic Index

Glycemic index is the rate at which a carbohydrate enters the bloodstream. The lower the glycemic index is, the more slowly it affects blood-sugar and insulin levels. Glycemic index is determined by the structure of the simple sugars, the fiber content, and the fat content. Understanding the glycemic index of your foods will help you manage your body's insulin production and minimize your tendency toward insulin resistance.

**The lower the number on the glycemic scale, the more slowly the sugar enters the bloodstream and the more consistent the delivery of glucose to your brain.**

100 = pure glucose

| | |
|---|---|
| High glycemic index | 70 and above |
| Medium glycemic index | 56–69 |
| Low glycemic index | Under 55 |

| Food | Glycemic Index |
|------|----------------|
| Oatmeal (rolled) | 22 |
| English Muffin | 11 |
| White bread | 14 |
| Whole wheat | 13 |
| Corn tortilla | 46 |
| White rice | 36 |
| Brown rice | 33 |
| White pasta | 47 |
| Whole wheat pasta | 37 |
| Orange | 42 |
| Banana | 25 |
| Apple | 15 |
| Pear | 11 |
| Carrot | 6 |
| Baked potato | 30 |
| Lentils | 18 |
| Cashews | 9 |
| Peanuts | 6 |
| Doughnut | 23 |
| Ice cream | 13 |
| Orange Juice | 53 |
| Bagel | 69 |
| Macaroni and cheese | 64 |
| Popcorn | 72 |
| Potato chips | 54 |
| Rice cakes | 82 |
| Raisins | 64 |

blood sugar rises. How high your blood-sugar levels go depends on what you eat, how much you eat, and how much insulin your body produces in response. Glucose then drops quickly and you have the urge to snack. Avoiding refined carbohydrates such as white rice and foods made from white flour will help to keep your blood-sugar levels optimal. Processed carbohydrates cause rapid and big increases in blood sugar. Eating whole grains, most fruits and vegetables, and beans produce gradual, smaller, and slower increases. The rule of thumb is that easily digested foods cause blood sugar and insulin to spike, which is a problem for HyperS, HypoP, and HyperP types.

How rapidly food is digested is affected by a number of factors. If grains are swollen, they are digested more quickly. The puffed rice in rice cakes has a higher glycemic index than brown rice. As we discussed earlier in this chapter, processing food often strips the outer, protective layer, which is hard to digest. The amount of fiber in food slows its digestion. For example, a whole orange with its natural fiber content will take longer to digest than will a glass of orange juice. Fiber that is indigestible carries partially digested food with it while passing through the intestines, so that food is not immediately digested. Food interactions also affect blood-sugar levels. Fat keeps food in the stomach longer, delaying its entry into the intestines. A food or meal that contains fat will keep blood-sugar levels down. This allows your body to maintain steady levels of sugar in your blood, keeping insulin production more steady and blood-sugar levels more consistent.

Remember, the "slower" the foods you eat, meaning the lower the glycemic index, the longer you will feel full. If you change the composition of your meals and snacks, you can lower your glycemic index. Eating fats at the same time as you eat carbohydrates will lower your glycemic index. **A combination of fat and protein with your carbohydrates will lower the index further.** For example, pasta has a glycemic index of 47, cheese ravioli is 39, and egg pasta 32. The plain pasta has no fat or protein, but the cheese and egg add fat and protein to the pasta, lowering the glycemic index because the protein and fat take longer to digest.

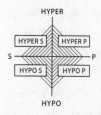

## OMEGA 3 FATTY ACIDS

After adipose tissue, your brain is the body part that contains the most fat. All the cells and organelles in your brain are very rich in polyunsaturated omega-3 fatty acids, also known as n-3 fats. These are essential fats, needed for normal functioning, and are derived from your diet. The omega-3 fats in our diets are ALA (alpha-linolenic acid), EPA (eicosapentaenoic acid), and DHA (docosahexaenoic acid).

ALA is the central omega-3 fatty acid in Western diets, found in vegetable oils, particularly soy, flaxseed, canola and walnut oil, eggs, leafy vegetables, wild game, and grass-fed animals. EPA and DHA are found in fish.

## THE BEST SOURCES OF OMEGA-3 FATTY ACIDS

Fish is the best source of EPA and DHA, but we urge you to be mindful of the toxic levels of mercury found in fish today. We recommend fish with the highest levels of fatty acids as a source for omega-3s. You should not eat more than two or three servings of fish a week. The fish to avoid, particularly for pregnant women, are shark, swordfish, king mackerel, tilefish, and tuna.

| EPA and DHA | ALA |
| --- | --- |
| Salmon | Flaxseeds |
| Mackerel | Flaxseed oil |
| Halibut | Canola (rapeseed) oil |
| Sardines | Soybeans and soybean oil |
| Herring | Walnuts and walnut oil |
| Anchovies | Pumpkin seeds and pumpkin seed oil |
| Oysters | |

If you are concerned about mercury and PCBs in the fish you eat or you simply don't like fish, you might want to try a fish-oil supplement. We recommend between 1000 and 2000 mg, depending on how much fish you eat.

The omega-3s are powerful protectors of your nervous system. DHA gives your brain cells the ability to transport nutrients into cells quickly and to remove debris and waste products. Omega-3s are anti-inflammatory, and they protect you from heart disease. Omega-3s are also essential for fetal-brain development.

There is an association between the drop in omega-3 fatty acids, particularly EPA, and the risk of depression. Studies have shown that as fish consumption goes up, depression rates go down. Ideally, we should consume equal amounts of omega-6 and omega-3 in our food. The typical Western diet includes fifteen times more omega-6 fatty acids than omega-3s, which is not good for your health. In the last several decades, our consumption of omega-3 fatty acids has declined significantly and been replaced with excessive amounts of omega-6 vegetable oils, such as corn and sunflower oils. In addition, food processing destroys omega-3 fatty acids to increase shelf life.

## EATING FOR OPTIMAL IMMUNE FUNCTION

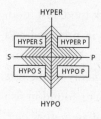

Your immune system is very sensitive to what you eat, and if your nutrition is not adequate, your immune system will be compromised. The major challenge for HypoSs and HypoPs is in their overly active immune system, which creates excess, damaging inflammation. Inflammation is the first response of your immune system to infection; damaging inflammation leads to asthma, allergies, and muscle and joint pain. The good news is that if you add the required nutrients to your diet, you will usually be able to restore immune function and reduce the inflammation that results from oxidative stress. It is extremely important for HypoSs and HypoPs to use nutrition to help to signal the immune system to calm down.

Oxidative stress occurs when the supply of antioxidants in the body is not sufficient to handle and neutralize free radicals, which are unstable molecules that interact aggressively with other molecules and create abnormal cells. This lack of balance results in massive cell damage that causes cellular mutations, tissue breakdown, and a weakened immune system. When free radicals are out of control, they accelerate aging and contribute to the development of cancer, Alzheimer's, Parkinson's, and cardiovascular disease.

In order to inhibit oxidative stress, quiet chronic inflammation, and promote optimal functioning of your immune system, your body needs essential amino acids, the essential fatty acid linoleic acid, vitamin A, folic acid, vitamins B6 and B12, vitamin C, vitamin E, zinc, copper, iron, and selenium. Deficiencies in one of more of these nutrients can affect your immune system and increase inflammation. When your body is inflamed on a cellular level, the aging process accelerates. Antioxidants are key to proper immune function; they calm the overly activated immune systems of HypoSs and HypoPs, and they boost immune function to help prevent colds and infections, which are major issues for the HyperS and HyperP types.

Some foods promote inflammation, including junk food, fast food, sugar, high-fat meats, saturated and trans fats used in prepared and processed foods, and nitrites found in hot dogs, some cold cuts, and sausages. A list of anti-inflammatory foods mirrors many of the lists we have given you in this chapter. Omega-3 fatty acids found in fish counter inflammation and are a key part of an anti-inflammatory diet.

## ANTI-INFLAMMATORY FOODS

**Vegetables:** arugula, asparagus, bean sprouts, bell peppers, bok choy, broccoli, broccoli rabe, brussels sprouts, cabbage, cauliflower, chard, collards, cucumber, endive, escarole, garlic, green beans, kale, leeks, mushrooms, onions, olives, romaine lettuce, scallions, shallots, spinach, sweet potatoes, zucchini.

**Fruit:** apples, avocados, blueberries, cantaloupe, cherries, clementines, guavas, honeydew, kiwifruit, kumquats, lemons, limes, oranges, papayas, peaches, pears, plums, raspberries, rhubarb, strawberries, tangerines, tomatoes.

**Animal proteins (grass-fed or wild preferred):** skinless and boneless chicken breast, turkey breast, anchovies, cod, halibut, herring, mackerel, oysters, rainbow trout, sablefish, salmon, sardines, shad, snapper, striped bass, tuna, whitefish.

**Nuts and seeds:** almonds, flaxseeds, hazelnuts, sunflower seeds, walnuts.

**Oils:** extra-virgin olive oil.

**Herbs and spices:** cocoa (70 percent cocoa), ginger, oregano, turmeric.

**Drinks:** Green tea, ginger tea, red wine (one glass a day).

HypoS and HypoP types need to incorporate these immune-calming foods into their daily diet, selecting foods from the lists in this chapter to have at every meal and every snack.

Now that you know the many beneficial effects of various nutrients, we hope you will be motivated to add those foods to your diet and to let your family know that healthy food is delicious food.

Stress only increases your need for a healthy diet, and we want you to understand the physical processes that are influenced by what you consume. When you become mindful about the foods you choose to eat, you will be more stress-resilient. You will also improve your mood, have more stamina and vitality, and prevent disease. The choice is up to you.

# CHAPTER SEVEN

# EXERCISE

Our research and experience with our patients has unquestionably demonstrated to us that increasing your physical activity is the most important thing you can do to combat stress and to age well. Exercise will refresh you by clearing your mind and calming your emotions. It improves the blood flow to your brain, supplying more energy for thinking and memory, and can put you in a mindset that promotes a more positive outlook on life. An active lifestyle will not only make you look and feel better, but your take on life will be more optimistic and you will experience an overall sense of wellbeing. Our goal in this chapter is to make you aware of how easy it is to improve your life by making physical activity just a small part of your day; just a half hour of moderate exercise most days of the week will have a powerful effect on your mind and body. Many of us spend more time than that on our hair and makeup every day. If you commit to exercise as a way of life, you will begin to feel and see the effects in just two weeks. Here are just some of the wonderful results that regular exercise can have in your life:

- losing weight, especially around the middle, and keeping it off
- looking and feeling younger
- boosting self-esteem

- diminishing stress
- alleviating depression and anxiety
- improving sleep
- building and maintaining healthy bones, muscles, and joints
- lowering the risk of developing heart disease, diabetes, high blood pressure, and cancer
- reversing or improving such life-threatening conditions

If scientists developed a medication that could deliver all these results, who wouldn't want to take such a powerful elixir? But, to produce those results, you have to get moving. According to *Newsweek* in 2007, only 31.3 percent of adults age eighteen years and older engage regularly in physical activity during their leisure time. More than 60 percent of Americans do not exercise on a regular basis, and 25 percent are not active at all. Fifty percent of young people, ages twelve to

---

### Real Life

Louise, age forty-two, is the primary breadwinner in her family. Though her husband tries to contribute, his efforts seem halfhearted to her. She has to take on the role of the CEO of the household as well. She had not been to see Beth since her third baby was born, four years earlier. She was embarrassed for missing so many of her annual visits.

Beth was surprised to hear that Louise had been struggling. She had chronic fatigue syndrome, likely the result of her stressful situation. She did not have the wherewithal to do what she had to do to stay on top of everything. A friend had motivated her to begin swimming in the neighborhood pool. She had been swimming nearly every day for close to four months. She swam slowly and deliberately, and it felt soothing to her. She was harsh in judging herself; she felt she wasn't swimming hard enough.

Recognizing Louise as a HypoP, Beth reassured her that working at a gentle pace was right for her and praised her for being so in touch with her body. Louise had begun to feel much better and her energy was returning. Her swimming had renewed her stamina and was having an impact on her stress response and her chronic fatigue syndrome.

twenty-one, are not getting the exercise they need on a regular basis. Physical inactivity has been linked to cardiovascular disease; hypertension; obesity; colon, breast, and prostate cancer; diabetes; and osteoporosis—all diseases that have been linked to stress. And inactivity leads to higher stress levels. The Centers for Disease Control and Prevention claim that physically active people have lower annual medical costs, fewer hospital stays and doctor visits, and use less medication than do inactive people. **Some scientists suggest that inactivity should be considered a disease state.**

> **From the Bench**
>
> **PHYSICAL ACTIVITY AS A NATURAL TRANQUILIZER**
>
> The strongest correlation between physical activity and psychological well-being is most pronounced with low to moderate physical activity—that's only two to four hours of walking per week. A study of 12,018 people found that those who made physical activity part of their leisure time were less prone to stress and feelings of dissatisfaction. Doesn't that seem like a minor time investment for such a big benefit?

Exercise can function as a positive coping strategy. When you approach exercise as an escape or a time-out from the problems and tensions of the day, exerting your body can be relaxing, a form of meditation. This removal from everyday tensions can go far to reduce stress. Having the discipline to exercise will give you a sense of control over your life and your body, and what could feel better than that in these frantic times?

## WHY EXERCISE REDUCES STRESS

Though physical threats are rare in our lives, emotional, social, or work stress evokes the same response: your body mobilizes energy to prepare you physically to confront or escape a threat, but psychological stress does not usually get solved quickly, nor does it require the increased metabolic demand it generates. The metabolic problems that result from the chronic activation of the stress response can develop into central obesity, hypertension, high cholesterol and triglycerides in the blood, and dysfunction in the cell walls, all of which can lead to metabolic syndrome and cardiovascular problems.

During your stress response there are more than fifteen hundred biochemical reactions. By-products of the stress response, like cortisol, continue to circulate in the body. You are already familiar with some of the harmful effects that can follow. Exercise removes the by-products of the stress response, because it provides the activity dictated by fight-or-flight. By using the energy produced by stress, physical activity allows the body to return to homeostasis faster and reduces the physiological impact of chronic, modern stress. In other words, since the stress response is a neuroendocrine mechanism that prepares the body for physical action, physical activity is a natural way to prevent the harmful consequences of stress by completing the process. Exercise can turn off or finish the stress response, and it's hard to think of a better coping technique than that. Exercise is particularly important for HyperS stress responders.

## A FULLER LOOK AT THE BENEFITS OF EXERCISE

- Exercise can provide an outlet for negative energy such as anger and hostility, which can make you ill if repressed. Physical exertion can be cathartic, releasing negative emotions in a healthy way.
- Exercise can increase your self-worth. You are choosing to do something that will help you and will alter your body image. High self-esteem has been shown to increase the ability to cope with stress.
- Exercise reduces muscle tension. Stressed muscles contract, known as "bracing," and lose their resting muscle tone. When you work your muscles, you release stored energy; then your muscles return to a normal resting state, which can reduce the aches and pains that bracing can produce.

- Exercise can be a moving meditation. Repetitive, consistent movement—found in swimming, skiing, jogging, biking—can alter your state of consciousness. The coordination of your breath with the movement is like a mantra. Exercise can create a state of tranquility and calm.

- Exercise can be an opportunity for social support. You might work out with a trainer, take a class, or have an exercise partner. By working out with others, you can satisfy your need for social support and expand your social network.

- You will sleep more soundly and experience less fatigue. An afternoon slump and evening exhaustion could be the result of inactivity instead of too little sleep. When you do aerobic exercise, your body transports and uses oxygen more efficiently to produce energy, and as a result you are slower to tire. In addition, moderate exercise three hours before bedtime can help you to relax and sleep better.

- You will become more in tune with your body. Exercise will increase your body awareness, enabling you to detect subtle changes that you were unaware of in the past. You will be able to recognize the physical effects of stress before damage is done. Women who are out of touch with their bodies have a hard time making the changes needed to remain healthy, while physically fit women can learn to relax more easily.

## PEARS OR APPLES ON THE MOVE

Where fat accumulates in your body is a good predictor of health. Pear-shaped women have deposits of fat primarily in their hips, thighs, and buttocks. Women who are HypoS types are more likely to be pear shaped. Apple-shaped women store fat in their abdomens. You do not have to be obese to have an excess of abdominal fat. Women of normal weight who store fat primarily in their bellies are at high risk for developing heart disease. Women who are HyperS types are more likely to be apple shaped even if they are lean.

To determine whether your abdominal fat is in the danger zone, you have to calculate the ratio of your waist to your hips. Measure your hips at the widest part of your buttocks, about seven inches below your waist. Take your waist measurement at the narrowest point, which is just above the navel. Divide your waist measurement by your hip measurement to get your waist-to-hip ratio. If the ratio exceeds .8, you are in the red-alert zone and should seriously undertake to reduce your belly fat. You can get a general sense of where you stand with just your waist measurement, but the waist–hip ratio is more accurate. If a woman's waist is larger than thirty-five inches, she is at the highest level of health risk.

Body mass index (BMI) is a significant measurement for obesity. To calculate your BMI, divide your body weight in pounds by your height in inches squared and multiply by 703, or check the table on pages 174–75.

According to the World Health Organization, a woman with a BMI more than 30 is considered obese, but BMI is not a universally accurate indicator. The percentage of body fat may differ based on sex, age, and fitness level. Women have a higher percentage of fat than do men at the same BMI, based on normal gender-based fat deposition. As we age, we lose muscle mass and have higher levels of fat. Very physically fit people—weightlifters, for example—have high levels of muscle mass, which weigh more than fat. If you have an excess of fat around your middle, as indicated by your hip–waist ratio, you face an additional health risk if your BMI is between 25 and 34.9 for developing type 2 diabetes, cardiovascular disease, high cholesterol, and high blood pressure.

If you are overweight or have an apple shape, it is time to focus

To use the BMI table, find the appropriate height (in inches) in the left-hand column labeled "Height." Move across to a given weight (in pounds). If you do not find your weight on the first table, please consult the second table, on page 175. The number at the top of the column is the BMI at that height and weight. Pounds have been rounded off.

| BMI | 19 | 20 | 21 | 22 | 23 | 24 | 25 | 26 | 27 | 28 | 29 | 30 | 31 | 32 | 33 | 34 | 35 |
|---|---|---|---|---|---|---|---|---|---|---|---|---|---|---|---|---|---|
| Height (inches) | Body Weight (pounds) | | | | | | | | | | | | | | | | |
| 58 | 91 | 96 | 100 | 105 | 110 | 115 | 119 | 124 | 129 | 134 | 138 | 143 | 148 | 153 | 158 | 162 | 167 |
| 59 | 94 | 99 | 104 | 109 | 114 | 119 | 124 | 128 | 133 | 138 | 143 | 148 | 153 | 158 | 163 | 168 | 173 |
| 60 | 97 | 102 | 107 | 112 | 118 | 123 | 128 | 133 | 138 | 143 | 148 | 153 | 158 | 163 | 168 | 174 | 179 |
| 61 | 100 | 106 | 111 | 116 | 122 | 127 | 132 | 137 | 143 | 148 | 153 | 158 | 164 | 169 | 174 | 180 | 185 |
| 62 | 104 | 109 | 115 | 120 | 126 | 131 | 136 | 142 | 147 | 153 | 158 | 164 | 169 | 175 | 180 | 186 | 191 |
| 63 | 107 | 113 | 118 | 124 | 130 | 135 | 141 | 146 | 152 | 158 | 163 | 169 | 175 | 180 | 186 | 191 | 197 |
| 64 | 110 | 116 | 122 | 128 | 134 | 140 | 145 | 151 | 157 | 163 | 169 | 174 | 180 | 186 | 192 | 197 | 204 |
| 65 | 114 | 120 | 126 | 132 | 138 | 144 | 150 | 156 | 162 | 168 | 174 | 180 | 186 | 192 | 198 | 204 | 210 |
| 66 | 118 | 124 | 130 | 136 | 142 | 148 | 155 | 161 | 167 | 173 | 179 | 186 | 192 | 198 | 204 | 210 | 216 |
| 67 | 121 | 127 | 134 | 140 | 146 | 153 | 159 | 166 | 172 | 178 | 185 | 191 | 198 | 204 | 211 | 217 | 223 |
| 68 | 125 | 131 | 138 | 144 | 151 | 158 | 164 | 171 | 177 | 184 | 190 | 197 | 203 | 210 | 216 | 223 | 230 |
| 69 | 128 | 135 | 142 | 149 | 155 | 162 | 169 | 176 | 182 | 189 | 196 | 203 | 209 | 216 | 223 | 230 | 236 |
| 70 | 132 | 139 | 146 | 153 | 160 | 167 | 174 | 181 | 188 | 195 | 202 | 209 | 216 | 222 | 229 | 236 | 243 |
| 71 | 136 | 143 | 150 | 157 | 165 | 172 | 179 | 186 | 193 | 200 | 208 | 215 | 222 | 229 | 236 | 243 | 250 |
| 72 | 140 | 147 | 154 | 162 | 169 | 177 | 184 | 191 | 199 | 206 | 213 | 221 | 228 | 235 | 242 | 250 | 258 |
| 73 | 144 | 151 | 159 | 166 | 174 | 182 | 189 | 197 | 204 | 212 | 219 | 227 | 235 | 242 | 250 | 257 | 265 |
| 74 | 148 | 155 | 163 | 171 | 179 | 186 | 194 | 202 | 210 | 218 | 225 | 233 | 241 | 249 | 256 | 264 | 272 |
| 75 | 152 | 160 | 168 | 176 | 184 | 192 | 200 | 208 | 216 | 224 | 232 | 240 | 248 | 256 | 264 | 272 | 279 |
| 76 | 156 | 164 | 172 | 180 | 189 | 197 | 205 | 213 | 221 | 230 | 238 | 246 | 254 | 263 | 271 | 279 | 287 |

on getting healthier. You should talk to your doctor about a program that's right for you, but getting healthier generally means combining good nutrition with physical activity to keep your chronic stress in check. **Exercise has a beneficial effect on how fat is distributed on your body by reducing abdominal fat and increasing lean body mass independent of weight loss.**

*To use the BMI table, find the appropriate height (in inches) in the left-hand column labeled "Height." Move across to a given weight (in pounds). The number at the top of the column is the BMI at that height and weight. Pounds have been rounded off.*

| BMI | 36 | 37 | 38 | 39 | 40 | 41 | 42 | 43 | 44 | 45 | 46 | 47 | 48 | 49 | 50 | 51 | 52 | 53 | 54 |
|---|---|---|---|---|---|---|---|---|---|---|---|---|---|---|---|---|---|---|---|
| Height (inches) | Body Weight (pounds) | | | | | | | | | | | | | | | | | | |
| 58 | 172 | 177 | 181 | 186 | 191 | 196 | 201 | 205 | 210 | 215 | 220 | 224 | 229 | 234 | 239 | 244 | 248 | 253 | 258 |
| 59 | 178 | 183 | 188 | 193 | 198 | 203 | 208 | 212 | 217 | 222 | 227 | 232 | 237 | 242 | 247 | 252 | 257 | 262 | 267 |
| 60 | 184 | 189 | 194 | 199 | 204 | 209 | 215 | 220 | 225 | 230 | 235 | 240 | 245 | 250 | 255 | 261 | 266 | 271 | 276 |
| 61 | 190 | 195 | 201 | 206 | 211 | 217 | 222 | 227 | 232 | 238 | 243 | 248 | 254 | 259 | 264 | 269 | 275 | 280 | 285 |
| 62 | 196 | 202 | 207 | 213 | 218 | 224 | 229 | 235 | 240 | 246 | 251 | 256 | 262 | 267 | 273 | 278 | 284 | 289 | 295 |
| 63 | 203 | 208 | 214 | 220 | 225 | 231 | 237 | 242 | 248 | 254 | 259 | 265 | 270 | 278 | 282 | 287 | 293 | 299 | 304 |
| 64 | 209 | 215 | 221 | 227 | 232 | 238 | 244 | 250 | 256 | 262 | 267 | 273 | 279 | 285 | 291 | 296 | 302 | 308 | 314 |
| 65 | 216 | 222 | 228 | 234 | 240 | 246 | 252 | 258 | 264 | 270 | 276 | 282 | 288 | 294 | 300 | 306 | 312 | 318 | 324 |
| 66 | 223 | 229 | 235 | 241 | 247 | 253 | 260 | 266 | 272 | 278 | 284 | 291 | 297 | 303 | 309 | 315 | 322 | 328 | 334 |
| 67 | 230 | 236 | 242 | 249 | 255 | 261 | 268 | 274 | 280 | 287 | 293 | 299 | 306 | 312 | 319 | 325 | 331 | 338 | 344 |
| 68 | 236 | 243 | 249 | 256 | 262 | 269 | 276 | 282 | 289 | 295 | 302 | 308 | 315 | 322 | 328 | 335 | 341 | 348 | 354 |
| 69 | 243 | 250 | 257 | 263 | 270 | 277 | 284 | 291 | 297 | 304 | 311 | 318 | 324 | 331 | 338 | 345 | 351 | 358 | 365 |
| 70 | 250 | 257 | 264 | 271 | 278 | 285 | 292 | 299 | 306 | 313 | 320 | 327 | 334 | 341 | 348 | 355 | 362 | 369 | 376 |
| 71 | 257 | 265 | 272 | 279 | 286 | 293 | 301 | 308 | 315 | 322 | 329 | 338 | 343 | 351 | 358 | 365 | 372 | 379 | 386 |
| 72 | 265 | 272 | 279 | 287 | 294 | 302 | 309 | 316 | 324 | 331 | 338 | 346 | 353 | 361 | 368 | 375 | 383 | 390 | 397 |
| 73 | 272 | 280 | 288 | 295 | 302 | 310 | 318 | 325 | 333 | 340 | 348 | 355 | 363 | 371 | 378 | 386 | 393 | 401 | 408 |
| 74 | 280 | 287 | 295 | 303 | 311 | 319 | 326 | 334 | 342 | 350 | 358 | 365 | 373 | 381 | 389 | 396 | 404 | 412 | 420 |
| 75 | 287 | 295 | 303 | 311 | 319 | 327 | 335 | 343 | 351 | 359 | 367 | 375 | 383 | 391 | 399 | 407 | 415 | 423 | 431 |
| 76 | 295 | 304 | 312 | 320 | 328 | 336 | 344 | 353 | 361 | 369 | 377 | 385 | 394 | 402 | 410 | 418 | 426 | 435 | 443 |

# WHAT IS MODERATE EXERCISE, ANYWAY?

Most of us overestimate how much exercise we get and underestimate how many calories we consume. For the purpose of stress relief, we are concerned about how much physical activity you get each day. At the start of your program, you should keep a record of the time of day you exercise, what you did, and how long you were physically active on the Stress-Detox Program Log. We recommend that the HyperS types exert themselves maximally to help balance their mobilized energy that needs to be put to use. HyperPs should exercise maximally, also, except for crash days. If you are a HypoS or HypoP, your constitution will not allow you to exert yourself as much. You should begin with light exercise and work up to moderate. It could be enlightening to record your mood and stress level before and after your workout. We have provided a space for that on the Stress-Detox Program Log on page 266.

## EXERCISE AND IMMUNITY

There is a link between regular physical activity and improved immune function. When you exercise, immune cells circulate more quickly through your body and are more powerful in destroying viruses and bacteria. A study of 547 adults between the ages of twenty and seventy at the University of South Carolina at Columbia examined the relationship between levels of activity and the risk of getting a cold. The participants who did moderate to high exercise four times a week had 20 to 30 percent fewer colds.

It's important to note that moderation appeared to be the key. Intense physical exercise may lead to a suppressed immune function that activates the stress response, and increased susceptibility follows. This reaction has been observed in marathoners, who often come down with a cold the week following the race.

## EXERCISE AND MOOD

Exercise activates serotonin and norepinephrine. When you are depressed, serotonin and norepinephrine are out of balance. Scientists believe that exercise might synchronize brain chemicals that affect mood. Inactive women are twice as likely to have symptoms of depression than those who are physically fit.

Exercise also stimulates endorphins, which create a feeling of euphoria or well-being, also known as "runner's high." Some feel that boost only twelve minutes into a workout. This boost can also reduce anxiety. One study found that walking was as effective as a tranquilizer in reducing tension, and the benefit lasted longer with exercise than it did with medication. The fact is that ongoing tension wreaks havoc on your self-esteem, one of the main sources of anxiety. Even people with depression generally feel less depressed after exercising for twenty to sixty minutes three or four times a week.

Physical activity may stimulate the growth of new brain cells that enhance memory and learning, both of which are negatively affected by depression. Scientists are now taking their research one step further

## From the Bench

### RECOVERING FROM MAJOR LIFE EVENTS

A study looked at one thousand college students following stressful events in their lives. Researchers found that subjects with high levels of aerobic fitness reported fewer physical health problems and less depression than those with lower levels of fitness. A high level of fitness was associated with reduced physiological response to laboratory stressors that required active coping or cognitive skills.

The researchers divided the group into three. For five weeks, one group received exercise training, one group had relaxation training, and one group had no treatment. The exercise group reported greater reductions in depression than did the subjects who had relaxation training or no treatment.

The differences diminished during the next five weeks, perhaps because of the general decline of depression over the time span, but the difference reemerged eight weeks later. The group doing exercise continued to show declines in depression. Aerobic exercise proved more effective than relaxation or no treatment following exposure to high levels of life stress, but after eight weeks, neither showed declines as significant as the group that exercised.

by studying whether regular exercise may reduce or even prevent the risk of developing depression.

## EXERCISE, CHOLESTEROL, AND BLOOD PRESSURE

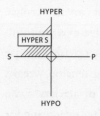

HyperS responders, with their elevated cortisol, are prone to having higher levels of harmful LDL cholesterol in the bloodstream and increased production of a precursor to triglycerides from the liver. Regular exercise reduces the amount of harmful, LDL cholesterol in the blood and increases the concentration of HDL, or good cholesterol. HDL helps to prevent clogging of blood vessels and is important for maintaining heart health. Walking eight to ten miles a week—an average of a little more than a mile, or about half an hour per day—may increase this protective form

### Real Life

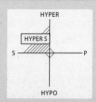

Cindy, who is fifty-nine, had a demanding job in marketing. Recently she had been putting on weight, particularly around her middle. She chalked it up to menopause. When she came in for her annual checkup, she was surprised to find that her blood pressure was high, at 150/90. When Stephanie saw Cindy's chart and asked her what was going on in her life, Cindy thought for a moment. Though she considered herself addicted to exercise, she realized she had been doing a minimal amount in recent months. She was working out with a personal trainer once a week at a gym and one-on-one with a Pilates coach one session a week, but she had been so busy at work, with so many pressing deadlines, that she had dropped her aerobic workouts on her home treadmill, preferring to spend the time with her family and friends. She had quickly lost the exercise habit.

Stephanie decided not to refer Cindy, a HyperS type, to her internist for blood-pressure medication yet. She recommended that Cindy get back to her aerobic workouts and invest in a blood-pressure monitor to keep track of how she was doing. She suggested that Cindy schedule a follow-up visit in a month so that they could study Cindy's blood-pressure readings.

Cindy began doing forty to fifty minutes on her treadmill five times a week, with a heart rate goal of at least 130. From the first day she went back to aerobics, Cindy's blood pressure returned to normal range.

of cholesterol. Exercise augments the ability of your muscles to take up and oxidize fatty acids and increases the activity of a lipoprotein, which makes the fatty acids of triglycerides available to muscle cells for energy metabolism. This action determines whether dietary fat or fuel mobilized during stress is for storage or for energy.

The MacArthur studies of successful aging found that low levels of physical fitness and high levels of emotional distress were associated with higher prevalence of metabolic syndrome compared with highly fit people. A two-and-a-half-year follow-up revealed that the inactive participants had high allostatic load, cardiovascular disease, and a decline in cognition.

## EXERCISE AND AGING—OR, NOW MORE THAN EVER

Physical inactivity can affect women more than men, because we have more body fat and less muscle and bone. As you age, muscle tissue and bone are lost. Since women have less to begin with, women are at greater risk at a younger age than men are for many problems associated with aging. Women may live longer than men on average, but our bodies will begin to fail us sooner. Regular exercise, no matter how old you are, can help preserve and improve flexibility, lung capacity, joint mobility, balance, posture, and stamina, and offers the cosmetic benefits of increased muscle tone and elasticity. If you are inactive, your muscles will become stiff and will sag from the pull of gravity. Your body will show signs of aging at an earlier age if you do not exercise.

According to the Mayo Clinic, many basic bodily functions start to decline at a rate of 2 percent per year after you pass age thirty. With exercise you can slow that decline to .5 percent per year. Women with little or no physical activity lose 70 percent of their functional ability by ninety; those who make physical activity part of their lives lose only 30 percent of their functional ability by that age.

If you do not get some form of exercise each day, your health will suffer. Women who are unfit tend to have greater HPA-axis reactivity to psychological stress as they age. One study found that white women age sixty-five and older who increased their activity to the equivalent of walking a mile a day lowered their risk of death in the six years following by between 40 and 50 percent. Running and brisk walking can counteract some of the negative aspects of aging and can add years to your life. Though strength training has not been shown to lengthen your life, that type of exercise improves your quality of life by providing you with the muscle power to perform everyday activities, allowing you to remain independent longer. Strength training is more important for aging women than for aging men because it increases muscle mass, preserves bone, and improves balance, all risk factors for

---

### Real Life

At her annual exam, June, a HypoP, complained that she ached all over. At seventy-eight, she feared that she was developing arthritis, but her internist had not found an obvious problem. Beth asked her about her nutrition, which was fine. June did say that she slept between two and three hours at a time at night. She would read and eventually fall back to sleep. She found herself taking quick naps during the day. Beth suggested that June begin a walking routine. June said she had never been one to exercise and dismissed the notion that she would start as she neared her eightieth birthday. Beth explained that moderate exercise could relieve the stiffness and achiness that was troubling June, and that her sleep could improve as well. June decided it was worth a try.

Beth recommended that June start by walking just ten minutes a day, preferably in the morning. June lived on Balboa Island, so she had easy access to the beach. Beth wrote out a plan for her to increase the length of her walks by ten-minute intervals weekly until she was walking forty minutes a day. She asked June to come back for a follow-up visit with a record of her exercise progress, including how she felt before and after exercise.

When June returned, she was up to forty minutes a day, which had made a big difference in her life. She was feeling better and sleeping very well. She had even made a new friend who was walking on the beach, too. They met every morning and walked together. June was sold on exercise and enjoyed the new friendship.

fractures, skeletal fragility, muscle weakness, and deteriorating balance, which are common in old age.

## ARTHRITIS, FIBROMYALGIA, AND CHRONIC FATIGUE SYNDROME

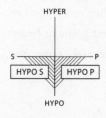

Many people over age fifty use the joint pain of arthritis as an excuse for limiting their physical activity. Aches and pains in your joints can make everyday activities difficult as you try to do everything from opening a jar or working at a keyboard. In particular, women suffering from fibromyalgia and chronic fatigue often feel that they hurt too much or do not have enough energy to exercise. HypoSs and HypoPs tend to develop these conditions, and are often unfit aerobically, with poor muscle strength and limited flexibility. The fact is that exercise is one of the most effective nonmedical treatments for pain reduction. If you have arthritis, consult your doctor before starting an exercise program, but by all means incorporate physical activity into your life.

Just like women with arthritis, fibromyalgia patients fear the pain of inappropriate exercise. For all these conditions, water-based exercise would be a good idea.

Intensity is what matters when you have pain and extreme fatigue. Exercise should be graded, starting with very low intensity. But the best way for you to get relief from these sometimes debilitating conditions is to become physically active. Exercise can combat your tendency for chronic pain by helping your body to produce endorphins, which are natural painkillers. If you have chronic fatigue, you might be able to handle only a few minutes of exercise a day. You might begin by just walking to your mailbox, doing some gentle stretches, or using two-pound arm weights as you watch TV. As exercise begins to feel easier, the duration can be increased gradually.

## THE GOOD NEWS FOR INACTIVE PEOPLE

In most studies, exercise had better outcomes for people who were more physically and psychologically unhealthy at the start of the studies. That means that it will be easier for you to see and feel positive results faster than you might believe possible. While it might be a hard adjustment for the first few days, you will start feeling more positive, more limber, and less pain after exercise. **The greatest gains in health occur when you go from an inactive lifestyle to a moderately active one.**

## ARE YOU READY?

By now, having absorbed all that physical activity can do for you, you must be ready to change into active wear and start moving to change your life. Remember, only thirty to fifty minutes of moderate activity most days of the week—that means five days—is all it takes to make a difference in how you feel. **According to the American College of Sports Medicine, you need to do only two and a half hours of moderate-intensity exercise per week to speed your efforts to lose weight.**

Yet starting to build more physical activity into your life can be daunting. There are always a million reasons not to exercise, the top one being that you just don't have the time. If you have any free time at all, you would rather spend it with your friends or family. Maybe you just don't like to exercise. You might tell yourself you are too out of shape, too old, too tired. You might be afraid of injuring yourself. Or you might feel self-conscious and decide that you want to lose weight before you begin putting yourself out there. To join a gym or buy equipment may seem too much of an investment. You might defeat yourself before you even begin, presuming that you will not be able to stick to it because it's too hard and you are not athletic.

Let's take a look at those excuses. You can certainly carve out some time on the weekend. Do you spend your leisure time during the week sitting in front of the TV, talking on the phone, or shopping online? Can you get up thirty minutes earlier in the morning? You don't have to do all your exercise at once. You can do ten-minute increments throughout the day. If you work, maybe you can have a brisk walk after lunch or before you start to prepare dinner. You could make it a family affair if you have children. Your entire family could enjoy a walk in the neighborhood after dinner. You could do a free-weight routine as you watch your favorite show on TV. If you are worried about cutting into time with family and friends, consider how much more you will be able to give others if you feel energized and upbeat. You could involve your friends in your program. Go for a bike ride instead of meeting a friend for a cup of coffee. Take a spin class together or play tennis at the town courts. Your body is meant to move. Regular exercise is not limited just to jogging, calisthenics, or weight training. You have to choose exercise that you enjoy doing.

For most people, the hardest part of adding physical activity to their lives is to begin. It doesn't take long to form a habit. If you commit to moving twenty minutes to a half hour five days a week, you will start feeling better in a matter of weeks. Moderate exercise can take many forms—and not all exercise is created equal in terms of how much time it takes to hit your goal. The more intensely you work out, the less time you will have to spend exercising. Shoveling snow for fifteen minutes is equivalent to walking for two miles in thirty minutes. Here are some examples of equivalent workouts:

15 minutes: climbing stairs or using a StairMaster, shoveling snow, jumping rope, biking four miles, running 1.5 miles
20 minutes: swimming laps, basketball
30 minutes: water aerobics, walking 2 miles, raking leaves, pushing a stroller 1.5 miles, aerobic dancing, biking 5 miles, shooting baskets

**Real Life**

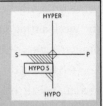

Pat was so overweight that she requested not to be weighed at her visits. On her chart, Beth estimated her weight at 250 pounds. Normally cheerful, Pat was worried about her health. At forty-three, her cholesterol was off the charts and her blood pressure was skyrocketing. Her internist had prescribed blood-pressure medicine and urged her to lose weight. Pat was mustering the will to join a weight-loss program that would help her improve her diet, but she was nervous about where to begin. Beth suggested that she add exercise to her program as well, explaining that exercise combined with good nutrition would speed up the process and make the results of Pat's efforts more dramatic. Pat protested: she felt too bulky and was afraid she would injure herself. If she hurt her hips or her knees, she wouldn't be able to move at all. Besides, she was self-conscious about how out of shape she was.

Beth suggested that she try water aerobics. Pat balked at the notion of being seen in a bathing suit in a public place. Beth suggested she work out at a quiet hour or join a class designed for weight loss. Pat found a gym near her home with an outdoor pool that was hardly ever used, giving her the privacy that she wanted. She was usually the only person in it and felt comfortable enough to start going through the exercises she had found online. One of the trainers at the gym helped her to develop a program. Her blood pressure and cholesterol began to drop, along with the weight.

After six months, Pat came in for a visit looking terrific. Each day, she would swim laps, do aerobics, or walk outdoors. She had made some exercise buddies at her weight-loss-program meetings. They all faced the same challenges and supported one another. Pat was elated to see her health and body return to the way they had been fifteen years earlier.

30–45 minutes: gardening, walking 1.75 miles (35 minutes)

45–60 minutes: playing volleyball, washing windows or floors, washing or waxing a car

## TAKING THE LEAP

Christopher Bergland, a world-class endurance athlete who has won the Triple Iron Man, the longest nonstop triathlon, three times, claims that it takes eight weeks for your mind and body to make the connection between moving and feeling good. Once that connection is made, you will associate exercise with pleasure, and movement will become a necessary part of your life. He says:

In order to muster the courage to get started, you always have to take a deep breath. Relax first. Commit to finish what you start. Lace up your sneakers and start today. Start now. Do something . . . do anything! Remember to take it slow. You don't have to kill yourself—getting the blood moving should be your goal. A small time commitment will reap huge benefits. As little as twenty to thirty minutes most days of the week is all you need to be doing to see results. That's less than 3 percent of your waking day, and you'll feel better for the other 97 percent. Think about it. Be pragmatic. That is a great return on investment.

—From *The Athlete's Way: Training Your Mind and Body to Experience the Joy of Exercise*

## AEROBIC V. ANAEROBIC EXERCISE

Aerobic exercise, meaning "with oxygen," involves rhythmic, sustained movement of low to moderate intensity for more than fifteen minutes. The idea is to get your heart pumping. In the next pages, we will show you how to calculate your heart rate and your maximum heart rate for exercise with goals for your type. Walking, using an elliptical machine, biking, swimming, and running all create a demand on the heart and lungs to deliver oxygen into the bloodstream. Aerobic movement derives energy from glucose and fatty acids, or stored fat from foods. Aerobic training stimulates the growth of capillaries, or small blood vessels, in your muscles that allow oxygen to be delivered more efficiently and lactic acid to be removed. **If your aim is to burn fat, workouts that are long, slow, and cover distances are the most effective.**

The health benefits of aerobic exercise include:

- Decreased body fat
- Lower resting heart rate
- Lower blood pressure
- Decreased LDL cholesterol
- Increased HDL cholesterol
- Increased life expectancy
- Some improvement in bone density
- Decreased stress

Anaerobic exercise consists of stop/start activities—short, intense bursts of activity, sometimes separated by periods of rest, like doing a weight circuit at a gym. You get anaerobic exercise when you sprint, lift weights, do competitive swimming, or play doubles tennis. Anaerobic exercise does not use oxygen to convert glycogen to energy; instead, the fuel is instantly available in the muscles and liver. The burst of activity communicates an immediate demand to the body. The most readily available form of energy comes from the glucose stores in the liver. This burst lasts only forty-five to ninety seconds. Another form of energy comes from creatine phosphate, a compound that is stored in the muscles. Anaerobic work burns only glucose, not fat or oxygen. It produces lactic acid, which is responsible for "the burn" you feel in your muscles after a hard workout. Lactic acid begins to accumulate when you exercise at 85 to 90 percent of your maximum heart rate, above the aerobic zone of 60 to 80 percent. Although anaerobic exercise does not burn fat, it creates lean muscle mass, which speeds up the metabolism, and that promotes more burning of body fat, not just during exercise.

The health benefits of anaerobic exercise differ from those of aerobic:

- Improved BMI
- Faster metabolism

- Stronger bones and connective tissue
- Prevents back pain and other injuries because muscles are strengthened
- Relieves stress

To gain and maintain fitness, many experts recommend two full body-strength-training workouts a week and at least three aerobic workouts. Some people combine their aerobic exercise with either upper- or lower-body workouts on consecutive days. You can combine aerobic and anaerobic work by hiking uphill or taking a step class, activities that require both quick, hard movements and sustained motions. You can add an anaerobic element to an aerobic workout by including some high-intensity intervals. Simply increase your speed and your heart rate for a few minutes. For example, if you are walking for thirty minutes, you might want to run or jog for three or four minutes, then return to a slower pace for five minutes, then run for three or four minutes. Adding a short high-intensity period can increase your strength and aerobic capacity, making you more fit. This is called interval training. Doing interval training can confuse your body and keep it from burning fewer calories by adapting to a steady pace or resistance.

## HOW TO CALCULATE YOUR MAXIMUM HEART RATE

The general formula for calculating your maximum heart rate is 220 minus your age. At a moderate level, you will be exercising at 60 to 80 percent of your maximum heart rate.

## HOW TO MEASURE YOUR HEART RATE

Turn one of your hands palm up and place the index and middle fingers of your other hand on your wrist below the base of your thumb or on the side of your neck. Refer to a watch or a clock with a second hand. When you feel your pulse, count the number of pulses in ten seconds. Multiply that number by six to get your heart rate per minute. Or you could count your pulse for six seconds and add a zero to the number. Your resting heart rate is taken in the morning before you sit up. The lower your resting heart rate, the better shape you are in. The following table will give you a sense of where you stand on the cardiovascular-fitness scale.

| Resting Heart Rate in Women | | | | | | |
|---|---|---|---|---|---|---|
| Age: | 18–25 | 26–35 | 36–45 | 46–55 | 56–65 | 65+ |
| Excellent: | 61–65 | 60–64 | 60–64 | 61–65 | 60–64 | 60–64 |
| Good: | 66–69 | 65–68 | 65–69 | 66–69 | 65–68 | 65–68 |
| Above average: | 70–73 | 69–72 | 70–73 | 70–73 | 69–73 | 69–72 |
| Average: | 74–78 | 73–76 | 74–78 | 74–77 | 74–77 | 73–76 |
| Below average: | 79–84 | 77–82 | 79–84 | 78–83 | 78–83 | 77–84 |
| Poor: | 85+ | 83+ | 85+ | 84+ | 84+ | 84+ |

To put this table in context, one study used data on 129,135 post-menopausal women enrolled in the Women's Health Initiative. It found that 20 percent of women had resting heart rates of 76 beats a minute or more and a 26 percent greater risk of heart attack in a follow-up period of nearly eight years.

Heart rate is one way to measure the demands you are putting on your body when you exercise. There is an easy way to measure how hard you are working with the Borg Rating Perceived Exertion Scale, in which you determine the intensity of your effort, the physical stress, and how tired you get while performing a physical activity. We've simplified the scale, which normally has twenty gradations, to five points.

# THE BORG RATING PERCEIVED EXERTION SCALE

1. **Very easy:** You can whistle a tune or sing a song. You are working out at 40 to 50 percent maximum heart rate. HypoPs should start here.

2. **Easy:** You can carry on a normal conversation. Your heart rate is 50 to 60 percent of maximum. HypoS types should start here. This should be the goal for HyperPs on a crash day.
   *Light exercise:* horseback riding at a walk; light stretching; bowling; golfing with a cart; walking slowly (1–2 mph); archery; billiards; croquet; playing the piano; fishing while sitting.

3. **Moderate:** You can speak short sentences of four to six words. Your heart rate is 60 to 80 percent of maximum. If you are a HyperS type, start your program at this intensity and work up. HypoSs and HypoPs should aim for this level on a regular basis.
   *Moderate exercise:* walking briskly (3–4 mph); pushing a stroller 1.5 miles in thirty minutes; swimming laps; canoeing/kayaking/rowing (2–3.9 mph); cycling (under 10 mph); dancing fast; golfing while carrying clubs; raking leaves; shoveling snow; skiing; leisurely ice skating; sailing; sledding; table tennis; belly dancing; calisthenics; aerobics class; hatha yoga, Pilates; aerobic dancing; working with light weights; power walking; virtual exercise with a video game.

4. **Hard:** You can get out two or three word fragments. You are working at 80 to 85 percent of your maximum heart rate. HyperSs should build to this level.

5. **Very hard:** You can nod your head, use sign language, and make unintelligible sounds. At this level, you are at 85 to 100 percent of your maximum heart rate. On a bad day, HyperSs can benefit from pushing their workouts to the max, if only for a few minutes.

   *Vigorous exercise:* mountain climbing; chopping wood; spinning; jogging (6 mph); jumping rope; surfing; playing singles tennis, racquetball, or squash; backpacking; ice skating or roller-blading; kundalini yoga; cross-country skiing; boxing; cycling (more than 10 mph); fencing; moving furniture; snow shoeing; kick boxing; soccer; walking briskly uphill while carrying something; lacrosse; field hockey; basketball; Bikram yoga.

As you become fitter, you will be able to challenge your body, but overdoing it at the beginning of your commitment will only undermine your efforts. Take it easy. You'll get as good a workout if you are willing to spend a bit more time.

## YOUR PLAN OF ACTION

As you think about beginning a program, consider your previous experiences. Did you join a gym near your office and never find the time to go? Was getting to the gym near your home too much of a production? Did you take a step class and find that unexpected events in your children's schedules kept interfering? Did you walk every day with a friend until it became unbearably cold? Did you have a routine that you just got bored with? If you can pinpoint what went wrong in the past, you might be able to avoid the pitfalls. However you decide to approach it, don't be too ambitious.

   If you know you will never drag yourself and your gear to a gym

## Real Life

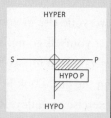

HYPER

S ——— P

HYPO P

HYPO

A close friend of Stephanie was very concerned about her sister, Charlotte, and asked Stephanie for advice. Charlotte was very isolated; she did not have friends and she did not date. She had worked in the same position for more than a decade and had rarely spoken about work or her colleagues. Her immediate family seemed her only social contacts.

Charlotte's sister was worried because, at age thirty-five, Charlotte had never had a mammogram. She agreed to make an appointment to see Stephanie since they had met socially several times before.

Charlotte was not very forthcoming during her visit to the office. Her responses to Stephanie's questions were flat and vague. It became clear that not only was Charlotte's social network practically nonexistent but she was also entirely sedentary. Knowing in advance that Charlotte was displaying the symptoms of a HypoP stress response, Stephanie had thought out a way to ease Charlotte from her shell. Stephanie told her that if she wanted more energy, she would have to expend some. She suggested that Charlotte take a short walk with her sister a few times a week, knowing that her friend would follow the prescription and make sure that Charlotte complied.

Stephanie's friend reported that they were walking regularly and that she had persuaded her sister to join her at her yoga stretching class. Charlotte seemed to enjoy getting in touch with her body and always left the class smiling. On her own, she signed up for a beginner's aerobics class. She started paying more attention to how she looked, and she was delighted when a group of women in her class invited her to join them for lunch. A woman from her yoga class invited her to attend a lecture given by a famous teacher. Charlotte was blossoming, and she had exercise to thank for it.

several times a week or you can't afford to join a gym, consider other alternatives: walk, do Pilates mat work with a DVD, or get a free weight program from a book or the internet and purchase inexpensive weights; three to five pounds would be a good start. Ease into your program; depending on your level of fitness, you might need to start with five minutes once or twice a day. You might begin by walking for ten minutes a day three times a week. If you add three minutes a week, you will be up to forty-five minutes in three months. There is no reason to rush. You have the rest of your life to improve.

If your schedule is demanding—and whose is not?—get up before everyone else in your house and have a quiet half hour to yourself to get yourself going. Exercising the first thing in the morning lifts your metabolism for six hours and will give you a surplus of energy to take on the day. Look at your schedule and try to carve out a time just for exercise each day. **Remember, you do not have to do your daily exercise in one shot. Three sessions of ten minutes will be just as effective as a single half-hour session.**

It is best to schedule a regular time for exercise, at least in the beginning. If you try to be flexible, you might find it too easy to put off your workout and end up skipping it. Some people choose to work with a trainer, even though it is costly, because they know they will show up for the appointment. But there is no reason why you cannot make an appointment with yourself. List your goals in your stress log and in your Stress-Detox Program Log so that you can reward yourself when you show progress. You might want to sleep better, lose weight, compete in a golf tournament, increase your running speed or distance, improve your tennis serve, or just feel better. You can keep track of your progress in your log. Evaluation of how you are doing will motivate you to keep going and to redefine your goals as you see the benefits of all your work.

## OVERALL EXERCISE TIPS

- To burn the maximum number of calories and fat, exercise on an empty stomach.
- For maximum performance, eat carbohydrates one hour before you exercise.
- Drink fluids—plain water is the best unless you are working out at high intensity or in extreme heat. In those circumstances you may require drinks with electrolytes.

- Exercising outside in the sun can improve your mood, especially if you have symptoms of depression.
- Exercising in bright light with an emphasis on duration rather than intensity will improve sleep, regardless of your fitness level.
- Running shoes are not forever. Depending on how hard you run, how long you jog, and how far you walk, they do wear out and give you less support, which can lead to stress injuries. Unless you are training for a marathon, a good running shoe should last six to eight months.
- Don't let travel interfere with your routine. Always pack your gym clothes, even on business trips. Many hotels have fitness centers or have arrangements with local gyms. If all else fails, you can take a long walk or jog in a local park.

You might want to build in some rewards when you have met a goal or reached a new level. Though a new outfit or a manicure is always a treat, focusing on things that will add to your enjoyment of your active time will reinforce your commitment. You could treat yourself to a pedometer, a wrist heart-rate monitor, a cute, comfortable outfit to wear when you exercise, a DVD of stretching exercises, a set of resistance bands, or an exercise ball.

Select activities that you enjoy doing. Physical activity does not have to be drudgery. If you find weight training torturous, ride a bike, play a sport, take ballroom dancing lessons, or even spend an afternoon planting some flowers. To keep yourself from getting bored, you can change it up by doing different things on different days.

Let your friends and family know about your commitment to change. They love you and will want to encourage you and support your efforts. It can be a big help to exercise with a friend or new acquaintance or to take a class. The social aspect of working out with a group or chatting with a friend while walking can have a double benefit in stress reduction, because you are satisfying a social need. If you spend time with people who are physically active, you are more likely to participate.

On the other hand, you might prefer to reserve your workout time for yourself. In a full and busy life, a solitary workout might be a minivacation, an oasis. Your friends and family will respect your need to regroup. If they do not, be firm in your resolve and explain your commitment convincingly.

## A VISIBLE, GROWING RECORD OF YOUR COMMITMENT

When you begin your program, buy a bag of rubber bands. Put a new rubber band on your wrist every morning or right before you exercise. It can serve as a reminder of your commitment. After your first workout, take that rubber band and tie it around itself to make the core of what will become a rubber-band ball. Every day you complete a workout, take the rubber band from your wrist and add it to the ball. You will watch that ball grow—a tangible reminder of what you have achieved.

"And you can bounce it around," says Christopher Bergland, who has used this technique in his own life and with the people he has trained. "Lifelong changes are made one day at a time. Recommit every day."

## QUIET THAT COMPLAINING VOICE IN YOUR HEAD

At first, adopting an active lifestyle can take discipline, but as you see and feel yourself transformed, you will actually look forward to your sessions. On those days when you are discouraged or when you feel it is too much effort, turn it around and look at the bright side. Instead of giving in to the whining voice in your head, be upbeat and cheer yourself on. Skipping your exercise when you are under stress is the worst thing you can do. In times of stress, you need physical activity the most.

## LOOK ON THE SUNNY SIDE

If you find that your negative thoughts are interfering with your ability to stick to your routine, try countering them with positive messages:

| Negative | Positive |
| --- | --- |
| I'm too exhausted even to think of moving. | I always have much more energy after I exercise. |
| I'm just so slow. | When I started I was winded so quickly. I may not be a speed demon, but I've really built up my endurance. |
| I've been doing this for two weeks. I just don't feel like it today. | Look at my rubber-band ball— it's already bigger than a ping-pong ball. I can't stall out now. |
| My whole body hurts from that last workout. | If I stretch well or take a hot bath, my muscles will be warmed up, and I'll be feeling no pain once I start moving. |
| I had to skip three days because I had a virus. It's always impossible for me to stay with it. Something always gets in the way. | Each day is a new day, and I can pick up where I left off. |

It's miserable out, so I think I'll just sleep in this morning.

It's raining too hard for me to enjoy my walk, I think I'll try that new yoga DVD.

This was the most stressful day at work in a long time. I think I'll make myself a martini.

I haven't been this stressed out in a long time. I bet a good workout will help me burn off this tension.

## ON YOUR MARK

In chapter 9, "The Stress-Detox Program for Your Type," we suggest the sort of exercise that will be most beneficial for stress relief for your type, but you have to experiment to find out what works best for you. Throughout this chapter, we have mentioned many different ways in which you can fulfill your very real need to exercise. In the end, if you don't enjoy your workout, you are putting a huge obstacle in your path to fitness. You and you alone are responsible for making exercise an enjoyable and satisfying part of your life.

We have not spelled out specific programs in this chapter because there is such a wealth of material available on fitness. Our goal is to inspire you to become more physically active by explaining the benefits and giving you the basics to gauge your level of fitness. Look at fitness magazines, books, websites, and try different things. There are entire programs online. Don't forget fitness shows on TV—try working out with different trainers that way. See what your local library has on fitness. Sign up for a trial membership at a health club and ask for help with the equipment. Take a class at the Y or local studios. Open your mind and explore. Think of developing a flexible program as an adventure. This is one commitment you will never regret.

# CHAPTER EIGHT

# RESTORATION

## Techniques to De-stress

The best defense against stress is a healthy lifestyle, which will make you more resistant to the daily pressures that raise your stress levels. You now have the basics on sleep, mental and emotional resilience, nutrition, and exercise. The final part of our program will provide you with a number of techniques that have been proven to help you relax and to restore your natural balance, which stress so dramatically disrupts. In order for your efforts to be most effective, you have to take a look at how you spend your time, how you interact with others, and what gives your life meaning and purpose.

Achieving a good work/life balance is a key element in stress reduction, and by work we do not just mean career. Running a household and raising a family are demanding jobs in and of themselves, and many working mothers juggle career and family responsibilities. But even if you are passionate about your work or are a veritable wonder woman, you still need time to yourself. If you don't take care of yourself, no one else will. Doing things just for yourself or having enjoyable hobbies will keep you vital, interested, and interesting. In this chapter, we will describe a number of restoration techniques. We make type-specific suggestions, but you have to experiment to decide what works best for you.

We are used to the protests of our patients when we give them this advice. They say, "There aren't enough hours in the day"; "I never stop racing from one thing to the next"; "I never have time for myself or my friends." As with exercise, you can begin with a modest time investment. When you begin to enjoy the benefits of these techniques, restoration time will become a much welcomed, necessary part of your day.

You need to take a close look at how you spend your time, especially if you feel you're about to spin out of control. Though most of us wish there were a few more hours in the day, learning time-management skills will go a long way to reducing stress and creating more time to do the things you enjoy.

## BE AWARE OF HOW YOU SPEND YOUR TIME

**Time-management experts suggest that you keep an activity log for several days.** Since you already have been using your Stress Journal for a number of different purposes, please add an activity log for a few days. If it's more convenient, you might prefer to carry a small pad or index cards for this purpose. Just record what you are doing every time you change activities. Not only will it help you to analyze how you spend your time, but the exercise will give you a sense of when you are the most productive during the day. Whether you are making your children's lunch for school while they eat breakfast, standing in line at a coffee shop for your morning coffee, getting in an early-morning run and then showering, or paying bills, just write it down. You should note changes in mood and energy at various times during the day, which will give you a concrete representation of your rhythms. At the end of the day, you will know the total amount of time you have spent on such activities as driving, cleaning, preparing meals, talking on the phone, and answering emails. From this log you will be able to indentify time wasters as well as develop a sense of when you are better fit to do specific tasks.

Keeping a monthly and a daily calendar will help you to stick to your Stress-Detox Program. Having the month laid out before your eyes, with doctors' appointments, social engagements, children's lessons, parties, athletic events, and deadlines will help you in planning a reasonably balanced schedule. On your daily schedule, which might be a pocket date book or an electronic version, make sure to schedule time for exercise and relaxation each day. If you block out that precious time in advance, you have a better chance of sticking to it. You can fill in the rest around it. It's time to put first things first.

## Real Life

Sara came to the office on the verge of a breakdown. She told Beth that her family was having financial difficulties. They were seriously overextended, and her husband's business was way off. Since he designed and installed kitchens and cabinetry, he viewed their home as a showcase, his calling card. Nearly everything they had was invested in that house. Struggling every month to meet their mortgage payments, they were about to hit rock bottom with their savings and didn't know where to turn. Her husband wanted Sara to ask her parents for a loan. Her parents had been generous to them over the years, but Sara could not see an end to their need, and, even if her parents bailed them out now, she and her husband would be back for help soon. Through all this stress and conflict, Sara had been struggling with chronic sinus infections, for which she was taking medication that knocked her out. She had been anxious and irritable and had not been sleeping. Beth told her that she had to start taking care of herself. Once she felt better, she would think more clearly and the answers would come to her. Beth recommended exercising regularly and adding fifteen minutes of mindful meditation to her day.

Sara called a few weeks later to say that she had taken Beth's recommendations to heart. She worked out at least five days a week, meditated, and prayed for a solution. She had realized that their expensive lifestyle had little to do with their happiness, and, although her husband was initially furious, she held her ground about approaching her parents. If they were living above their means, it was time to make a change.

They put the house on the market, and because it was such a show place, it sold quickly despite the poor housing market. They found a simple cottage, which they bought outright. As the cloud of anxiety and stress lifted, Sara's husband thanked her for her common sense and firmness. The entire family was happier and looked forward to having a cozy time together in their new home.

# YOU GET TO PICK THE A-LIST

All of us have an endless to-do list, and facing all we feel we have to do can be overwhelming. The way to avoid that buried-alive feeling is to assess what you have to do and to prioritize, so that you have an efficient plan of action. As you look at your list, select the tasks that must get done that day or week or that seem much more important than other chores and activities on your list. These high-priority items become your A-list. If you prioritize what you have to do and have a rolling list, you will get a lot accomplished. And you might discover that some things you assume you have to do can be eliminated. On the flip side of that, it is fine to say no if your plate is full. Most of us have the tendency to take on too much, and saying no can make us feel selfish and guilty. **The truth is that you don't have to accept every invitation you receive or do everything your family, friends, boss, and colleagues ask of you.** If you are overextended and overcommitted, be pleasant and firm as you set your boundaries. The ability to say no without feeling guilty will protect you from overload.

# STREAMLINE YOUR LIFE

Being disorganized creates stress. Disorder wastes time and causes frustration. **Your life will run more smoothly if you simplify.** In the United States, we tend to own too much. In recent history, houses kept getting bigger—more rooms and walk-in closets to fill. The financial crisis has given everyone pause, reminding us that there is a limit to what we need. It's time to make your life less complicated.

Start small—not with the attic or basement, which in many homes can be the most daunting areas to tackle. Instead, choose a place that needs organizing—your clothing drawers, the linen closet, the kitchen cabinets, the toys. Make piles of things you definitely want to keep, rejects, and maybes. If the rejects are in good condition, you could give them to a member of your extended family, a friend, or a charity. Be tough in going through the "maybe" pile; chances are you would not miss an item, and the likelihood is that you will never use it. If a dress has sentimental value but really does not fit anymore, take a picture and then give it away. All you really need is the memory. There is no reason to clutter your life with things you do not need.

As you get the hang of clearing things out, you can tackle the bigger jobs, perhaps with the help of your partner or an objective friend. There is nothing like pristine surfaces and empty space in your cabinets, drawers, and closets to make you feel unencumbered and light. Imagine being able to put your hands on anything you want immediately, without having to take the time to search. That could be a significant stress reducer.

Some people have a system of getting rid of something when they buy something new. The idea is to buy and accumulate less. **Buy only what you need, and when you do, buy only what you love.** That way you will surround yourself with things that make you happy and please your senses.

## THE IMPORTANCE OF CONNECTION

One of our central themes in this book is that humans are social by nature. Your brain works in a way that reflects the world and people around you. Even more important for women, the tend-and-befriend response to stress causes you to seek social support. **When you make a positive social contact, your opioid pathways kick in, and your stress response is quieted.** You could volunteer to work in a soup kitchen or with the elderly. Helping those less fortunate than you is one of the best ways to counter stress. You are fulfilling a real social function when you do so.

In addition to giving emotional support, friends and advisers can

### Real Life

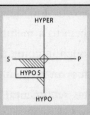

Janine, a twenty-six-year-old junior high teacher, a HypoS responder, came to see Beth a number of times because she had debilitating headaches at the time of her period. Her mother often came with Janine to the appointments and would barely let Janine speak. She was overbearing, correcting anything Janine tried to say. It was clear to Beth that this had been a lifelong pattern. She wondered if Janine had any independence or if her mother controlled every aspect of her life, including her friends.

Beth ran a number of tests that showed nothing was physically wrong with Janine. Janine's mother called almost daily to get the results and was told by our staff that they could release the information only to Janine. Her mother went ballistic and threatened to show up at the office herself. Beth called to let Janine know that the tests did not show anything physically wrong with her. When Janine apologized profusely for her mother's out-of-control behavior, Beth asked her to make another appointment to talk about the results and to decide on a course of action. Beth dreaded the show-down that would occur when Janine came with her mother.

Beth's surprise was evident when she found Janine alone in the examination room. Janine beamed and said that she had refused to let her mother come to the appointment and had not even told her when it was scheduled. She said that her mother had crossed the line when she made such a scene about the test results and Janine had had to take a stand. She was tired of her mother's meddling in her life and felt as if a huge burden had been removed from her shoulders.

Beth reviewed the test findings with her and suggested that Janine take some Pilates classes and try either progressive muscle relaxation to relax the tension that was so visible in her body. Beth recommended that she lean on her best friends for support during this difficult time as she was trying to restructure her life to decrease her mother's influence. She reminded Jeanine of how physically and emotionally beneficial female emotional support can be. A follow-up visit three months later revealed an almost miraculous improvement.

help you appraise a situation, avoid stressful situations entirely, or deal with negative consequences. They may have information or a point of view that provides you with new insight. People whom you trust can assist you in dealing with negative emotions and can help you to step back from your problems and view them with more objectivity. Your social network can provide you with guidance and expand your resources. All this makes being in the world easier and more satisfying. Isolation kills the human spirit.

## QUICK FIXES FOR CALMING DOWN

When you feel tied up in knots, you can do many things to relax. The few restoration techniques we provide in this chapter have been tested by researchers, but there are many other ways you can take a break to calm down. Our patients have contributed to this list to give you an idea of the quick fixes that work for them. Use your imagination and indulge yourself.

Take a bath with scented oils
Get lost in a good book
Try a new recipe
Take a nap
Watch a chick flick
Take your dog for a long walk
Find water—a beach, lake, river, pond, or stream
Pick fruit
Talk to a stranger
Plant a windowsill herb garden
Dance
Clean and organize
Look at puppies and kittens in a pet store
Go to a country fair or street fair
Spend time in a bookstore or library
Go window-shopping
Go to a wine-tasting

Plan a minivacation
Go to bed early
Explore classes you could take
Do a crossword puzzle
Volunteer
Buy fresh flowers
Go bird watching
Flip through a magazine
Organize your photos
Catch up with an old friend
Go antiquing
Have a cup of tea
Listen to great music
Call a friend
Visit a botanical garden
Exercise
Give yourself a facial
Go to the zoo
Help someone
Look at art in a book, gallery, or museum

Go for a mani/pedi or do it
  yourself
Sing
Make a date to meet a friend
Play with your children
Go to a park
Sit in a café and people-watch
Have a news blackout
Go to a church or temple
Join a group
Light a scented candle
Sit on a park bench

Let a makeup artist at a
  department store give you a
  complimentary makeover
Explore a new neighborhood
Go to a farmers' market
Walk in the rain
Plan a party
Sunbathe (with sunblock)
Rock in a rocking chair
Play a musical instrument
Laugh or cry
Be grateful

You get the idea. There are countless things you can do to lift your spirits and defuse your tension. Be good to yourself. Not only do you deserve it, but you need it.

> **Warning**
>
> It is essential for you to consult with your doctor if you have hypertension, cardiovascular disease, diabetes, epilepsy, or psychiatric problems before trying the following techniques.

## CALMING BREATH

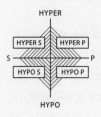

This is a fundamental relaxation technique that all stress types should practice. You have probably taken a deep breath before plunging into something—a difficult conversation, serving a tennis ball, trying not to cry. When you sigh, you are unconsciously using a relaxation technique by inhaling more air than usual

> **Three Types of Breathing**
>
> **Upper costal breathing** involves the upper third of your chest, moving primarily the intercostal muscles that connect the ribs. This is very shallow, rapid breathing. This happens when tension levels rise, and the muscles in the abdomen tighten.
>
> **Thoracic or middle costal breathing**—normal breathing involves the middle third of your chest, from the sixth rib down.
>
> **Diaphragmatic breathing** expands the belly and moves the diaphragm. Breathing from your abdomen reduces stress and induces a state of quiet and calm. Deep breathing involves your entire chest.

and exhaling. Deep breathing has a calming and centering effect, and you can do it anyplace, anytime for a quick fix for acute stress.

The most obvious role of breathing is to supply your blood with oxygen and to dispel carbon dioxide. The passage of air is also important for communication. Without air passing through the lungs, you would not have a voice, nor could you smell anything. Since the passage of air is important to your ability to express yourself, breathing difficulties may signify difficulties in social interaction and experience.

Breathing is often an indicator of how you feel. When you are relaxed, your breathing is most likely steady, even, and involves your diaphragm and even abdominal muscles. When you are upset or stressed, your breath becomes shallow, irregular, and quick. This sort of breathing involves only the top part of your lungs. Breathing therapy has been used successfully with a number of stress-induced conditions, including simply feeling tense, concentration problems, headache, chronic fatigue, and burnout. Deep breathing can relieve symptoms of depression, panic disorder, phobia, and anxiety. The practice of deep breathing has been shown to ameliorate neck, shoulder, and lower-back complaints, chronic pain, shortness of breath, and stuttering. In addition, heart disease, asthma, COPD, and neurological diseases, including Parkinson's, respond well to this technique.

# HOW TO DO DIAPHRAGMATIC BREATHING

## LYING DOWN

- Lie flat on your back on a mat or towel on the floor. Make sure your head is well supported.
- Place a book on your belly.
- Inhale counting 1, 2, 3, 4, 5, and watch the book rise.
- Exhale counting 1, 2, 3, 4, 5, and watch the book fall.

## SITTING UP

- Sit comfortably in a straight-back chair with your feet on the floor.
- Put your right hand on your abdomen; your hand should be pushed out by your belly as you inhale and fall as you exhale.
- Count on the inhalation and exhalation, if you like.

Just watch out for hyperventilation: if you breathe too deeply or too rapidly or practice deep breathing for too long, you risk hyperventilating. This condition results from reduced carbon dioxide in the blood, which causes constriction of the blood vessels in your brain. When you hyperventilate, the pH balance in your blood becomes more alkaline, which leads to nerve and muscle excitability. If you experience any of the following symptoms while practicing deep breathing, breathe less deeply or more slowly or stop entirely: dizziness, faintness, blurred vision, cold hands or feet, shivering, cramps, tightness in your chest, hot flashes, headache, stiffness around the mouth, sweating, a warm feeling in your head, rapid heartbeat, blurred vision, tension, panic, and surreal feelings.

# MEDITATION

Meditation is one of the most popular restoration techniques, because you can learn it quickly and incorporate it easily into your daily life. The practice of meditation is a structured, effective way to use your mind to relax your body. By withdrawing your senses from life's demands and what is distracting or troubling you, you gain control over your attention.

When Herbert Benson and his colleagues studied the effects and processes of meditation on the relaxation response, they found that two elements were required: a mental device and a passive attitude. A mental device could be a sound, word, mantra, or prayer that is repeated silently or chanted aloud. It could be visual—gazing at a single object, like a painting, for example. A passive attitude has to do with emptying your mind of distracting thoughts in order to regain your mental focus. You can evoke the relaxation response even while working out at a noisy gym as long as you stay focused and are able to keep other thoughts from intruding.

Meditation puts you in a rare state of fluid consciousness that has qualities of sleep and wakefulness not unlike the hypnagogic state of falling asleep. EEGs of meditators have shown patterns of high alpha- and occasional theta-wave patterns and swift shifts from alpha to sleeplike frequencies. During meditation you will enter a state of profound physiological relaxation that resembles the deepest nonrapid-eye-movement sleep, but this happens while you are awake.

People who meditate regularly claim that they become more productive and report being better able to cope in high-stress jobs. Many experience a surge of energy after meditating, increased stamina, and greater creativity. Meditation may allow you to weaken your habitual reactions and experience only natural, moment-to-moment responses to situations. You're more efficient and don't waste energy by calling upon old habits to respond to new circumstances.

Meditation improves your ability to regulate your emotions and to slow down your reactions. You will learn to tolerate stress and to resist cravings rather than respond impulsively; meditation also interrupts the flow of negative thinking. Meditating can free you from patterns of avoidance and attraction that have driven you for your whole life. Going within can change your eating behavior and food choices as your awareness of hunger, satisfaction, and emotional eating gets deeper. Some studies of Tibetan monks have shown that meditation can enhance activities in areas of the prefrontal cortex that underlie positive emotions. Doesn't all of this make you want to start right now? But there is more.

Though the study of meditation in the United States focuses on secular meditative practice, meditation has always been a traditional part of religious training. Practitioners achieved inner peace, transcendence, and sometimes mystical experiences. On a spiritual level, you will grow to understand that you are separate from your thoughts. This heightened self-awareness will lead you to self-acceptance. Harsh self-judgment and ruminative thinking is at the core of the stress response, and meditation is a potent restoration technique. If you are more compassionate with yourself, that generosity will carry over in your relationships, enhancing the social support so necessary to everyone's well-being.

There are many different forms of meditation, but we are going to focus on just two general types, mantra and mindfulness meditation. Mantra meditation focuses your attention, because you repeat a word or phrase in your mind or focus on something unchanging. Mindfulness meditation is nonconcentrative. In other words, you shift your focus and attention to the world around you and passively "watch" it go by. When you practice this sort of meditation, you open yourself up and expand your field of attention to include as much mental activity as possible. Whichever kind works best for you, meditating will make you more aware of your inner processes. Since you remove yourself from being in the world, meditation creates a richer understanding of your inner self. If you adopt the practice, you will develop a new kind of communion between you and your self.

## MANTRA MEDITATION

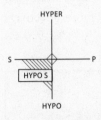

Mantra meditation uses a sound as its focus. Many people think of saying the word *Om* during meditation, but any word would work. Herbert Benson used the word *one* in his studies. Transcendental Meditation assigns you a personal mantra to use, but you can use anything as a mantra. You can also just focus on your breathing and say, "In, out" in your mind. Your mantra doesn't even have to mean anything. It can just be a sound. Whatever you choose, repeat your mantra in your mind and make it tie to your breathing. If your mind wanders from your mantra, bring your attention back to it. Do not judge yourself. Direct your attention back to your mantra in a gentle, easy manner. Wave goodbye to that thought in your mind.

For many people, mantra meditation is easier to learn than mindfulness meditation. The mantra works as a distraction from the incessant flow of thoughts, sensations, and emotions that fill your mind. We recommend this type of meditation for HypoS types to free the mind of draining thoughts and to renew energy. Over time, your mantra will become a signal to turn inward. The rhythmic repetition of a mantra acts as a natural tranquilizer, and the word itself will act as a trigger for the state of relaxation that is associated with your meditation. The permissive attitude with which you let thoughts, images, or sensations flow through your mind without rejecting or attaching to them will create a rich subjective state.

Many people who meditate report a feeling of freshness when they finish meditating and a heightened awareness when they return their attention to the world, making them highly receptive. They claim that colors are brighter, sound is clearer, and all their senses are sharper. You will be quickly reviewing a broad range of speculations, memories, emotions, and concerns in a state of deep relaxation. The soothing effect of the rhythmic repetition of your mantra can neutralize disturbing thoughts. The rhythm will connect you to deep biological rhythms, stabilizing you and allowing you to deal more effectively with the external environment.

---

### Balancing Your Brain Hemispheres

Brain imaging has shown that the workload of the cerebral hemispheres can be equalized through meditation. Normally, the left hemisphere dominates your thinking, almost to the exclusion of the right. When you meditate, the activity of the left side of your brain, which is verbal, linear, and time linked, decreases, while the right side of your brain, which is wordless, intuitive, and holistic, becomes more dominant. There is a shift in the balance of power between the hemispheres. This occurs when you are new to meditation. When you become more advanced, the activity of the two hemispheres reaches a balance, maximizing your brain power all the time.

---

## MINDFULNESS MEDITATION

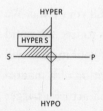

Popularized by Jon Kabat-Zinn, a professor of medicine at the University of Massachusetts, mindfulness meditation is a passive meditation. Rather than focus on a single object, you meditate on the moment-by-moment flow of whatever crosses your mind or intrudes from the environment. You pay attention to each moment and the stimuli that come and go. Mindfulness is a focus on the here and now, paying attention to what is, without being judgmental. Your awareness is broad and fluid, and you avoid being analytical. This calms the brain and body by stopping the flood of thoughts that often provoke or prolong stress.

We are not used to thinking like this; our minds are always active, busying themselves with a steady stream of consciousness. The Buddhists refer to this intense self-talk as our "monkey minds," that chattering and jumping around that goes on inside our heads all the time. Your goal in mindfulness meditation is to observe where your monkey mind wants to lead your attention but not follow it. Just observe the thoughts that stream through your mind without responding to them. If a police car goes by on the street with sirens blaring, think, "A police car is going by." Simply acknowledge what your senses have experienced. While meditating, you attempt to develop a stable, nonreactive awareness of what is going on in your environment and of your thoughts, feelings, and senses. This type of meditation works well for HyperS women. It will keep your mind from racing and will help to alleviate some of your anxiety.

To practice this type of meditation, observe where your attention is. Are you planning or worrying? Are you thinking about what happened yesterday or years ago? Do you feel good, neutral, anxious, or sad? Is your body tight or relaxed, your breath deep or shallow? Do you smell the scented candle you have lit? Do you feel relaxed in the chair in which you are sitting? Is your jaw tense? When you are mindful, you become a mirror that reflects your internal and external world without comment.

Do not be surprised if your inner life is chaotic. As you observe what floats through your mind, you begin to discern certain patterns and learn to pay attention without engaging or reacting. You might think of being angry about something your partner did, but you stay separate from the emotion and do not feel the same stress that you might when not meditating. While meditating, you suspend your reactions. As you do so, you begin to learn viscerally that most physical and emotional experiences are transient; those reactions tend to be knee-jerk reactions, not well-contemplated, necessary responses. As you get in the habit of disengaging repeatedly, your mind will create different patterns of responding. Instead of reacting automatically, you will have the chance to use more-integrated responses. You will see that you have control over how you react to things. Just as in cognitive therapy, you will be able to change your conditioned, knee-jerk responses. Not reacting in set ways to the noise from your "monkey mind" will give you a sense of freedom.

## THE MECHANICS OF MEDITATION

In time, you will be able to meditate anywhere, but as you begin to learn how to meditate, you should find a quiet place to avoid distractions. Wear comfortable clothing that doesn't bind or itch. You should attempt to meditate twice a day for ten to twenty minutes, ideally before breakfast and dinner. Do not meditate for too long. Overdoing it can have a detrimental effect, because difficult emotional material can sometimes arise.

If you have a problem sitting still for that long, as a HyperS might, meditate for as long as you can. Start with just three minutes if you need to; forcing yourself to be still and meditate is counter to what you are trying to achieve. You might want to try taking minimeditation breaks every other hour. You can do three-minute or five-minute mini-meditations anytime you are stressed.

Do not meditate after meals, because your blood is pooled in your stomach to aid digestion. Try not to drink a caffeinated beverage or smoke a cigarette before meditation, because you don't need extra stimulation when you are trying to relax. The technique may enhance the action of certain drugs, specifically antianxiety, antidepressant, antihypertensive, and thyroid. The dosage should be monitored by your physician. Sometimes the dosage can be lowered or even discontinued as a result of your practice, but that has to be determined by a doctor.

You can look at a watch or clock placed near you if you are uncertain how much time has elapsed. Or, you can set a timer or alarm—just make certain that the alarm is not too harsh. A quiet tone from your cell phone would work. It will not be long until your natural clock will bring you back to normal consciousness at the right time.

## HOW TO MEDITATE

1. Sit erect in a comfortable chair with your hands in your lap.
2. Allow your body to be still. Feel as if you are sinking into the chair. Close your eyes. Take two or three diaphragmatic breaths. Notice your increased sense of calm.
3. Begin to breathe naturally. Feel the air enter your nose, move through your throat, and enter your lungs as your stomach expands and falls back again.
4. If you are doing **mantra meditation,** begin to repeat your mantra silently. Do not focus on the noises, thoughts, concerns, and feelings that flow through your mind. If you get caught up in a thought or sensation or noise, observe it and push it away, returning to your mantra. Do not criticize yourself if you lose focus. Continue this way for the session.
5. You focus on your breath in **mindfulness meditation.** As your "monkey mind" serves up thoughts and feelings, try to let them pass without reaction. Just observe the thoughts as they come and go as if you are watching a movie. Let the ideas and images pass on by.
6. You might remember something from the past or think about the future. If you become distracted by a thought, just observe it and understand that it is the habit of your mind to pursue the thought. When this begins to happen, gently turn your attention away from the thought and return it to your breathing.

7. When you mind wanders off, do not be critical of yourself. The mind becomes attached to everyday concerns, feelings, and plans for the future. When your mind rests on a thought, do not pursue it. Return your focus to your breathing.

8. **If you are uncomfortable, dizzy, or experience disturbing images or hallucinations, open your eyes and stop meditating.**

9. When you are ready to end your session of meditation, first return your attention to your breath. Then bring your attention back into your body and the room. Move around gently in the chair. When you are ready, open your eyes and stretch out.

# YOGA

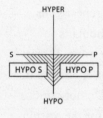

Yoga is a physical and mental discipline that was developed thousands of years ago in India. The word *yoga* is derived from the Sanskrit word *yuj*, which means to control, yoke, or unite. The practice of yoga is designed to direct and concentrate your attention and to develop mental and physical health, inner harmony, and a communion between you and a universal, transcendent existence.

In the most general terms, the practice of yoga will improve your body awareness, decrease your heart rate, calm you down while stimulating you, enhance relaxation, and help you to center. The claims for yoga's effects on health are too numerous to list. You can practice yoga just for the exercise, without a spiritual intent, and you can pursue the peace and calm that is at the heart of the yogic philosophy. Yoga is excellent for HypoSs and HypoPs. Improved flexibility and blood flow will help your aching muscles.

Though there are many branches of traditional yoga, we in the West tend to be most familiar with hatha yoga, which consist of a series of positions that stretch and relax the body. In Bikram yoga and other "hot" yogas, positions are held in a set order in a very hot room, allowing your muscles to stretch easily. Hot yoga is a very challenging workout and is not for everyone.

There is much material readily available on yoga, so we will not go into this restoration technique in great detail. The practice of yoga has become part of our culture. You can go online to read about it. There are numerous yoga magazines and thousands of books, CDs, and DVDs available. In any city or town, there are yoga teachers and studios. Classes are offered at gyms, community centers, senior centers, and adult extension courses. You might want to try a class with a friend or go on your own to meet a new group of people. The privacy of your home might be more calming for you, though it is good to have a teacher's guidance as you learn the positions. There is nothing like starting the day with a Sun Salutation, a series of positions that gets your juices going.

## PROGRESSIVE MUSCLE RELAXATION

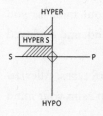

In 1905, Edmund Jacobson studied the startle reaction to unexpected loud noise. In what was the first systematic study of relaxation, he was intrigued to find that relaxed people had no obvious startle response to sudden noise. He went on to study knee-jerk reflexes, finding that the amplitude of the response was lower with relaxed subjects. When electromyography (EMG) was developed, he was able to measure muscle tension directly. That is when he made a major breakthrough, discovering that just the thought of moving an arm or a leg was accompanied by an EMG response in that limb. If you were to think of knocking on a door twice, there would be two unique EMG bursts in that arm.

Jacobson and his colleagues observed that when we encounter a stressful situation, our bodies react reflexively with a primitive star-tle pattern. We rise on the balls of the feet and hunch forward. This posture can be actual or it can be internal, marked by tension in the muscles. The entire musculoskeletal system reacts within one hundred milliseconds, preparing the body for fight-or-flight. Increased muscle tension triggers a burst of sympathetic activity, causing a constriction of blood vessels within the muscles. The stress response is in play. Chronic and excessive tightening of the muscles puts the central ner-vous system into overdrive, which increases the activity of the auto-nomic nervous, cardiovascular, and endocrine systems.

Progressive muscle relaxation involves tensing a set of muscles and then relaxing them. The technique works on the idea that once you can identify the sensation of tension, you can relax it away. The tech-nique enables you to identify a specific tense place, and then you relax that spot. You observe the difference and apply it to all your muscle groups. The technique is like internal biofeedback, a process we will discuss later. By practicing this technique, you will learn automatically to be aware of tension in your body and to release it. Relaxing your muscles reduces the activity of your HPA axis and the excitability of your sympathetic nervous system. You will relax your mind as you relax your body. **Relaxed muscles mean a relaxed mind, and a relaxed mind means relaxed muscles.**

This technique is highly recommended for HyperS types. Alleviat-ing your generalized muscle tension can actually help calm your mind as well as lower your muscle pain and tension.

## THE GOAL OF PROGRESSIVE MUSCLE RELAXATION

Jacobson created progressive muscle relaxation to help people become sensitive to what is going on in their bodies. It is a method designed to heighten your internal observation. Just as cognitive therapy gives you the tools for psychological introspection, progressive muscle relaxation provides you with a means for physiological introspection. By practicing this technique, you will learn to recognize states of tension in your body. It does not require a big time investment; three daily practice sessions of just five minutes each can have a significant effect in a few weeks' time.

> **If you have high blood pressure, we advise you to try a different relaxation technique. The contractions required in this method can raise systolic blood pressure. After you have lowered your blood pressure with other techniques, you can try this one.**

## HOW TO DO PROGRESSIVE MUSCLE RELAXATION

Practice progressive muscle relaxation in a warm, quiet room. Muscles do not relax as efficiently in cooler environments. It is best to do this technique before eating, so that your blood flow is not directed to your digestion. When first learning the technique, lie on the floor so that your muscles are completely supported. If you prefer, you could use a reclining chair. Let your arms and legs go, rotating out. Place your hands on your stomach or at your sides. Make yourself comfortable. You might like to use a small pillow under your neck or knees. As you get more proficient, you can do the exercise while sitting or standing.

Progressive muscle relaxation deals with sixteen muscle groups. You will focus first on your hands and arms, starting with your dominant hand—that is, most of us would start with the right side. If you are left-handed, begin on your left side. You will move to your face, neck, and down your body to your feet. The first step of the technique is to contract a given muscle group, producing a good deal of tension. You then release that tension all at once, creating a momentum that will cause the muscles to relax more deeply. You will relax as much as you tense, like a pendulum swinging from side to side. Your relaxation will be deeper because of this momentum, compared to just relaxing the muscles without tensing first.

The following lists will take you through the movements in order and explain the best way to tense each muscle group.

## THE SCRIPT FOR PROGRESSIVE MUSCLE RELAXATION

### PUTTING IT TOGETHER

Progressive muscle relaxation is very straightforward. There are only a few steps:

- Take a deep breath and hold it before you tense.
- When you contract a muscle group, focus all your attention on those muscles.
- Tense the muscle group with as much force as you can. Hold the contraction for about five seconds.
- Notice the tightness and what tension feels like in those muscles.
- Let all the tension go.
- Notice the pleasurable sensation in those muscles. Breathe slowly for thirty to forty seconds.

Repeat the process with the same muscle group. Then move on to the next part of your body.

| Muscles | How to Tense |
| --- | --- |
| 1. Right hand and forearm | Make a tight fist with your upper arm relaxed. |
| 2. Right upper arm | Press your elbow down against floor or chair. |

| Muscles | How to Tense |
|---|---|
| 3. Left hand and forearm | Same as # 1 |
| 4. Left upper arm | Same as # 2 |
| 5. Forehead | Raise your eyebrows as high as possible. |
| 6. Upper checks and nose | Wrinkle your nose and squint your eyes. |
| 7. Lower face | Clench your jaw and smirk. |
| 8. Neck | Try to raise and lower your chin at the same time. |
| 9. Chest, shoulders, upper back | Take a deep breath, hold it, and pull your shoulder blades together. |
| 10. Abdomen | Try to push your stomach out and pull it in at the same time. |
| 11. Right upper leg | Simultaneously contract the large muscles on the front of your leg with the smaller ones underneath. Press your heel down on the floor. Flex your foot, pointing your toes toward your head. |
| 12. Right foot | Point your toes, turn your foot in, and curl your toes gently. |
| 13. Left upper leg | Same as # 11 |
| 14. Left calf | Same as # 12 |
| 15. Left foot | Same as # 13 |

You can do spot checks on your tension level during the day. If your neck and shoulders are tense or ache after reading a presentation at the office, you can reduce that tension by lifting your shoulders up to your ears and relaxing them several times. You might hold tension in your core region, holding your stomach muscles rigidly. Pull those muscles in even more tightly, pressing your lower back to the chair or the floor. If you are standing, tilt your pelvis forward. Then release your stomach muscles. If you realize that you are breathing shallowly, you can press your shoulders back to expand your chest and inhale deeply. If you are grinding your teeth or furrowing your brow, you can work on your face. Where you hold tension will be different for each of you. When you have time to do the full progression, you will be able to measure the level of relaxation you achieve in trouble spots as compared to other areas. This is how you train yourself to melt tension from your body, which will stop your muscles from sending stress signals to your brain and will extinguish your body's stress response.

**Body scanning** is a technique with which you do a spot check on your body. Even when you are tense, some part of your body is relaxed. After you learn progressive muscle relaxation, you will be able to locate a relaxed area and to spread that sensation to the rest of your body. You can visualize that relaxed feeling as a ball that travels to different parts of your body to warm and relax them.

## AUTOGENIC TRAINING WITH GUIDED IMAGERY

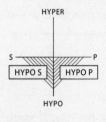

Autogenic training is one of the oldest relaxation techniques, used widely in Europe, Russia, and Japan, but less popular in the United States. In 1900, Oska Vogt, a brain physiologist, discovered that people could put themselves into a hypnotic trance and produce the sensations of heaviness and warmth in the limbs at will. This technique is best for the HypoS and HypoP types. It will help you alter autonomic dysfunction by promoting balance between the sympathetic and parasympathetic systems. The sensation of heaviness results from the relaxation of muscles and warmth from the dilation of blood vessels, which creates increased blood flow. He found that those subjects experienced less tension, fatigue, and fewer headaches than other patients. Johannes Schultz, a German neurologist who practiced psychiatry, synthesized his clinical experience with hypnosis using Oska Vogt's observations in brain research to create autogenic training.

Autogenic training taps in to the self-healing and self-regulatory powers of the body, linking the mind and the body, promoting homeostasis and the knowledge that we can learn to regulate this built-in mechanism. Autogenic training is bi-directional, working not only to reduce excessive autonomic arousal but to raise low levels of automatic function. Self-hypnosis, a form of passive concentration, like meditation, enables you to achieve deep relaxation.

You can use guided imagery to individualize the technique. Imagine a calm, soothing setting when you need to reduce your extreme stress sensitivity, and imagine exciting or motivating experiences when you need stimulation due to your fatigue. You do not try to do anything. You simply focus on inner sensations as you do the exercises. Meditation uses the mind to relax the body; autogenic training uses the sensations of heaviness and warmth to relax the body and then extends the relaxation to the mind by employing imagery.

Those who suffer chronic pain have been shown to tolerate pain better when they practice autogenic training. The psychological effects can be very powerful. The reduction of anxiety, depression, and fatigue have all been associated with this method. In general, those who regularly practice autogenic training raise their stress tolerance.

**Warning: If you have psychiatric problems, your autogenic training should occur in a clinical situation with trained clinicians. Talk to your doctor.**

# THE MECHANICS OF AUTOGENICS

To become proficient, you need to practice ten to forty minutes, twice a day. It could take as much as several months of regular practice to become accomplished at this technique, but resist the urge to push it. Your body will respond on its own timetable, so be patient. You can practice autogenic training in three postures: lying down, seated erect, and seated relaxed. Here are the specifics:

**Lying down:** lie on your back with your feet slightly apart, falling slightly to the outside. Use cushions wherever you need to make your body comfortable. Make sure you are in alignment. Place your arms next to your torso, but not touching your body, with a slight bend in the elbows. Keep your hands palms up. This is the preferred position because the neck is well supported.

**Seated erect:** sit on a high-backed chair that will align your head with your torso. Sit back in the chair so that it supports your thighs. Rest your arms on the sides of the chair or keep them in your lap.

**Seated relaxed:** use a low-backed chair or a stool with no back support. Sit forward on the seat, feet placed at shoulder width. Lean forward and support your arms on your thighs. Let your hands and fingers dangle from your knees. Drop your chin to your chest, head hanging loosely.

Select a position that works for you. Your aim is for your body to be as relaxed as possible, with no muscle contractions. The exercise is done with your eyes closed.

# THE SCRIPT FOR AUTOGENIC TRAINING

There are six stages of this training:

1. Focus on a sensation of heaviness in each arm and each leg (start with your right if you are right-handed, left if you are left-handed). Begin with each arm, followed by each leg.
2. Focus on the sensation of warmth in each arm and each leg.
3. Focus on the calm and regular beating of your heart.
4. Focus on your breathing, which will come naturally on its own.
5. Focus on warmth in your abdomen.
6. Focus on coolness in your forehead.

You will have to prepare a script for yourself. Until you learn it, it might be more relaxing to tape your voice reciting the instructions or to have someone read them to you. Of course, CDs are available to help you. There is a logic to the flow of these exercises that should be easy to learn. The script should go like this:

1. My right arm is heavy (repeat six times).
2. My left arm is heavy (repeat six times).
3. I am very quiet (one time).
4. My right leg is heavy (six times).
5. My left leg is heavy (six times).
6. I am very quiet (one time).
7. My right arm is pleasantly warm (six times).
8. My left arm is pleasantly warm (six times).
9. I am very quiet (one time).
10. My right leg is pleasantly warm (six times).
11. My left leg is pleasantly warm (six times).

12. I am very quiet (one time).
13. My heart is beating calmly and regularly (six times).
14. I am very quiet (one time).
15. It breathes me (six times).

Within eight weeks you will be able to produce these sensations voluntarily and will achieve a state of deep relaxation in a few minutes. Do not be alarmed if you experience a tingling sensation in your arms and legs: the engorgement of blood in your limbs can create pressure on the nerves in your arms and legs.

## BENEFITS OF AUTOGENIC TRAINING

Autogenic training affects sympathetic tone and parasympathetic activity. As with other relaxation techniques, this method reduces heart rate, respiratory rate, cholesterol level, and muscle tension. Studies have shown this technique to be effective for those who suffer insomnia, migraines, and high blood pressure. Numerous studies have shown that autogenic training has a positive effect on the following conditions: lower-back pain, asthma, diabetes, ulcers, hemorrhoids, indigestion, constipation, and tuberculosis. Those who suffer chronic pain have been shown to tolerate pain better when they practice autogenic training. The psychological effects can be very powerful. The reduction of anxiety, depression, and fatigue have been associated with this method. In general, those who regularly practice autogenic training raise their stress tolerance.

## AUTOGENIC MEDITATION OR IMAGERY

If you want to take your relaxation deeper, you can use imagery to relax your mind even more, after you have gone through the autogenic script. All you have to do is keep your eyes closed and roll your eyes upward as if you are looking at your forehead. You might want to start by visualizing a color, then colors combining to make a picture. Then imagine a single object against a dark background and focus on that. Now you are ready for some imagery work.

One effective exercise is to imagine yourself in a relaxing scene. Maybe you are floating in aquamarine Caribbean waters, feeling the hot sun on your skin as the waves lap gently on the brilliant-white crescent beach. Maybe you are walking through a field of colorful, fragrant wildflowers with butterflies fluttering around you. You could be snuggled under a cashmere throw in front of a blazing fire while a blizzard storms outside. Maybe you have just finished a splendid meal served on a terrace overlooking a vineyard as you watch an awe-inspiring sunset.

As you imagine the scene, observe the minutest detail. How does the air feel? What are the colors that surround you? Can you hear the wind howling outside, birds flying overhead, or a babbling stream? Can you smell the crackling fire or the bouquet of a rich burgundy? How do you feel? Use as many senses as you can to imagine the scene. You will transport your mind from routine cares.

If you want to increase your insight, you could visualize yourself in various emotional states in different situations. You could imagine yourself floating on a cloud and letting your anxiety drift away. You could see yourself completing a challenging project and being praised by your boss. Or you could use imagery to envision someone with whom you are in conflict from a neutral point of view to gain insight about the root of the conflict. The therapeutic uses of imagery are endless if you are creative and relaxed about the process.

# BIOFEEDBACK

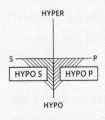

Biofeedback trains you to use signals from your body to improve your health. The technique gives you the awareness of bodily functions and the possibility of controlling those functions consciously. Employing instruments to measure various functions, including blood pressure, heart rate, skin temperature, sweat-gland activity, and muscle tension, you learn what is happening in your body and how to control it. Just as progressive muscle relaxation allows you to identify how your body feels when your muscles are tense, biofeedback uses external instruments to measure different parameters in your body so that you can recognize how internal imbalance feels and how it differs from the feeling of being in balance. If you can create warmth and heaviness in your body when you practice autogenic training or reduce your blood pressure by meditating, you can gain control of many physical processes that used to be considered automatic responses. The technique familiarizes you with the sensations of relaxation and measures your particular physical correlates, giving you a numerical picture of how your body operates in a relaxed state.

A complex pattern of oscillation occurs in your body at all times. Your heart rate, blood pressure, body temperature, and available energy, along with your mood and attention, are never stable. Science has made sense of the variability that might seem chaotic and has discovered that patterns constitute the body's self-regulatory reflexes. When the body is well regulated, the oscillations are of high amplitude. If the amplitude of the oscillations is reduced, it is a sign of vulnerability, indicating that the body's self-regulatory mechanisms are damaged or not working well and cannot handle stress, injury, or disease. Biofeedback is designed to measure these oscillations and to enable you to restore your self-regulatory mechanisms. Your goal is to be able to control your heart rate, the dilation of your blood vessels, the conductance of your skin, brain waves, muscle tension, blood pressure, and the secretion of hydrochloric acid in your stomach.

The instant gratification of the biofeedback process is motivating.

## THE BENEFITS OF BIOFEEDBACK

The training can measure how certain mental states affect your body. By getting a direct reading of how your feelings and thought processes are reflected by your body functions, you can focus your attention on mental states that you need to alter for your health. You can use your ABCDE log (see chapter 2) to work on your attitudes and emotional reactions.

Biofeedback has been found helpful for the following conditions: asthma, insomnia, sweaty palms, excessive snoring, temperomandibular disorder, attention deficit hyperactivity disorder, leg-muscle weakness, and incontinence. On a psychological level, biofeedback helps with phobias, anxiety, stage fright, depression, alcoholism, drug abuse, psychogenic cough, and burnout.

Biofeedback is believed to have an even more global effect. If you learn that you have control over systems in your body you never believed possible, you just might be able to control other areas in your life that you are completely in charge of, such as eating well, exercising, and regularly restoring yourself. This process might well inspire you to make better choices for your health.

Since HypoPs are out of touch with their bodies and are in an extreme state, biofeedback is an important option for them. It is the most efficient way to reconnect with what it feels like to be back in balance and gives you the power to control your response.

## WHERE TO FIND BIOFEEDBACK EQUIPMENT

Though biofeedback equipment that works with a home computer or laptop is available, it is expensive. You can check with a local hospital or the psychological-counseling or health-education departments of a nearby college or university to see if they have biofeedback programs. There will be psychologists in your community who work with biofeedback as well. Inexpensive courses may be offered at an adult extension course, spa, or town center. If you offer to participate in research at a hospital or university, you might be able to learn the technique and get paid for it instead of paying. Though you do have to go to the trouble of finding available equipment and someone to train you, biofeedback is a very efficient technique, and you will see its results quickly.

## MASSAGE, REFLEXOLOGY, AND ACUPRESSURE

A great massage is an enjoyable and effective way to relieve your stress. Massage helps to relieve muscle tension and stiffness, provides great joint flexibility and range of motion, alleviates discomfort during pregnancy, reduces formation of scar tissue, pain, and swelling, enhances athletic performance, improves blood circulation and movement of lymph fluids, reduces blood pressure, helps relieve tension headaches and the effects of eye strain, enhances the health and nourishment of the skin, improves posture, strengthens the immune system, and helps with rehabilitation after surgery or injury.

Massage therapy is the manipulation of soft tissues of your body to produce effects on your muscles, veins, and nerves. A massage therapist can feel where your body is holding stress and work it out. A one-hour massage can have an effect similar to that of many sessions of progressive muscle relaxation. There are many forms of massage therapy, including:

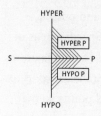

**Swedish massage,** developed by Per Hendrik Ling in the eighteenth century, uses long strokes, kneading, and friction on the muscles and moves the joints to improve flexibility. This type of massage is best for HypoPs to improve circulation to their aching muscles and joints. HyperPs will be revitalized by a Swedish massage on their crash days.

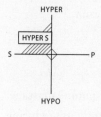

**Deep tissue massage** employs patterns of strokes and deep finger pressure on muscles that are tight or knotted, focusing on muscles deep under the skin. This type of message will relieve HyperSs of their deep-seated muscle tension and will alleviate mental tension as it does so.

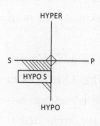

**Pressure-point massage** uses different strokes with deeper, more focused pressure on the trigger points, or knots, that can form in the muscles and be painful when pressed, causing symptoms elsewhere in the body. HypoSs should consider this to alleviate the trigger points in their inflamed muscles.

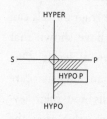

**Shiatsu massage,** a traditional Japanese technique, involves varying, rhythmic pressures on the acupressure meridian points in your body. This will benefit HypoPs by balancing their disrupted, desynchronized systems.

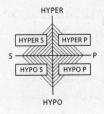

**Reflexology** focuses on massaging and putting pressure on the soles of your feet. Specific areas of the foot are believed to correspond to organs or structures in the body. The goal of reflexology is to clear blockages in these organs and points so that energy, or the life force, can flow freely through your body. Reflexology is beneficial for all types. Your feet are rich in nerve supply, and massaging your feet stimulates the release of oxytocin and the calming effects that result.

## THE BENEFITS OF MASSAGE

Studies have shown that following a twenty- to thirty-minute massage, cortisol levels and heart rate can be reduced significantly. By reducing anxiety, massage can enhance your capacity for calm thinking and creativity. When you are stressed out, a massage can satisfy the need for a caring, nurturing touch that is not sexual.

Massages are often enhanced by aromatherapy, an added touch that can be relaxing, invigorating, and stress reducing. Oils derived from plants with medicinal qualities can be mixed with massage oils to add fragrance and additional benefits to your massage. Some herbal essences can heal wounds, fight infections, assist in blood circulation, and aid digestion, because the healing properties of the plants are absorbed into the bloodstream. Of course, these fragrant oils can be infused in the air you breathe as well. Studies have shown that lavender and rosemary essential oils decrease cortisol levels. One study showed that aromatherapy and massage in an intensive-care environment significantly improved patients' moods and their levels of anxiety. They reported feeling much more positive after the therapy.

If you want to splurge, treat yourself to a massage at a day spa. Maybe you can find a massage school in your area that needs bodies on which students can practice. Or you might consider having a spa night at home. You and your partner can learn massage techniques from a book or DVD. It could do a lot for your relationship.

---

**Massage and Modesty**

If you have never had a massage and have modesty issues, you might be more comfortable with the idea if you understood that the massage therapist works one limb at a time, with the rest of your body covered. While you are on your stomach, the towel is lowered to your waist so that your back can be massaged. That is the most exposed you ever are. While you are lying on your back, only your face, head, shoulders, and limbs are worked on. The rest of you is modestly covered by a towel.

---

## QIGONG AND TAI CHI

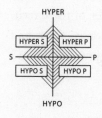

*Qigong,* which is pronounced "chee gong," is a term used for a number of ancient, traditional Chinese energy exercises and healing practices. The practice begins with guided physical movements that require concentration and promote the qi energy flow in the body. The controlled, nonimpact movement is gentle.

The practice is said to improve many stress-related conditions, including allergy, asthma, hypertension, premenstrual syndrome, insomnia, headache, back or neck pain, addiction, depression, and anxiety. We think all types would benefit from this ancient technique, which combines almost all the other techniques and works on many systems in the body at once. People who practice qigong claim that their lives are improved in significant ways. They report a more harmonious state of mind and body. They feel less stressed, their ailments are improved, they resist illness, and they become more sensitive to their bodily processes. They develop the ability to regulate their own health and vitality. Though qigong may seem esoteric, we mention it here because it combines so many of the techniques we have discussed in this chapter: relaxation, breath work, guided imagery, slow movement, biofeedback, mindfulness mediation, and mind/body integration.

Tai chi, developed in China hundreds of years ago, is a form of martial arts, using exercise, relaxation, breathing techniques, and meditation. The philosophy of yin and yang—opposing forces—is the fundamental principle of tai chi. Tai chi consists of slow, graceful movements and shifts of balance that look like dance combined with meditation and breath control. The aim is to integrate your mind and body.

We have a tall stack of studies that show tai chi is a very powerful stress-reduction technique. Several studies found that tai chi may have benefit in preventing or treating cardiovascular disease and increases bone density, agility, and flexibility.

Though qigong and tai chi are not as popular in the West as yoga is, it could be worth your while to investigate if either of these techniques would work for you. A large selection of books, CDs, and DVDs is available. Both qigong and tai chi are taught in studios all over America.

# JOURNALING

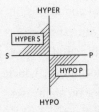

Journaling is very important for HypoPs. You can use journaling to connect your feelings to your physical expressions of emotions. The process is a private, nonthreatening way to learn how to connect to your emotions. In time, you may be able to express more of yourself verbally. Journaling has been shown to alleviate pain for HypoPs.

For HyperSs, who tend to be anxious, with thoughts racing through their minds, journaling can quiet the mind. Recording your concerns at a given time each day could help to clear your mind and help you sleep.

Keep a notepad next to your bed so that you can jot things down when you wake up during the night with something on your mind.

Journaling, the process of describing your reaction to an event, an emotion, or a worry, can take the sting out of negative emotions and give you insights into what you are experiencing, especially if you employ one of the relaxation techniques described in this chapter before you begin to write. Writing about your deepest thoughts and feelings about traumatic events or just bad experiences can improve your mood, give you a more positive outlook, and improve your health.

Sit at your computer, or pull out a piece of paper or a beautiful notebook you use just for this purpose, and write about an event, memory, or thought that disturbed you. It could be something trivial, like someone cutting in front of you in line or a more significant event like finding out your teenage son had been drinking at a party. Just describe the event, how you felt, how you handled it, and whether the resolution was satisfying or requires more from you. Now and then, remember to write about something that made you happy or for which you are grateful. Though describing and expressing how you feel about a negative event can increase your understanding and be a relief, writing about something positive can amplify your feelings of well-being. When something wonderful happens, get the most from it.

## From the Bench

### WRITING IT DOWN CAN HELP

One study of forty-seven women who had been abused randomly assigned some of the women to four writing sessions in which they were asked to focus on traumatic life events or a neutral topic. They found that depressed women who were assigned to write experienced a drop in their depression symptoms. The researchers concluded that expressive writing could reduce depression. Another study of participants with elevated blood pressure found that systolic and diastolic blood pressure decreased significantly in the group assigned to expressive writing.

Writing about frustration, anger, despair, doubt, envy, or worries can force you to clarify your feelings and to release them. You can write whatever you want without fearing the judgment of someone else. The effort can distance you from those negative feelings, and the process can help you put whatever happened behind you and keep the situation from having continued power over you. Expressing what you feel is a way to dissolve your stress and to restore yourself.

## SPIRITUALITY AND PRAYER

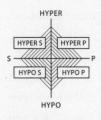

Spirituality is many things to many people, but whatever form it takes, spirituality gives life meaning. In the broadest sense, spirituality is the search for the sacred in life, for experiences and values that are transcendent. For some, spirituality involves living according to a religious doctrine that fosters

**Real Life**

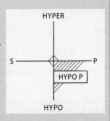

Hannah's ulcerative colitis had intensified. Her bouts were becoming more frequent and extremely painful. Hannah did not talk very much, rarely smiled, and seemed to have shut down emotionally. She told Stephanie about the worsening of her condition during a recent visit. Stephanie never felt she got to know Hannah very well. She knew from her chart that she was forty-eight and married, but that was it. Stephanie was sure that she was observing a symptom of a HypoP stress type and told Hannah that it might help if she kept a journal. She advised Hannah to record how she felt when she began to experience cramps in her abdomen. Stephanie suggested that, in time, Hannah might see a pattern or a connection between what she was thinking and feeling and flare-ups of her colitis. Verbalizing these feelings could become an outlet for them. Hannah looked skeptical but agreed to give it a try.

A few months later, at her annual checkup, Hanna thanked Stephanie warmly for her advice. Journaling had made her aware of her tendency to suppress her emotions. Having expressed her feelings on paper, the feelings eventually dissipated. Her colitis was under better control.

spiritual experience. Belief in God or a higher power can make our concerns seem less urgent in the scheme of things. Others define the spiritual quest as finding their purpose in life. Everyone wants to learn how to create more love, joy, peace, fulfillment, and connectedness. Some want to commit themselves to continued growth, to achieving their full potential. Spirituality can also be about living in the moment, being mindful of every aspect of existence. Spirituality encompasses all these things and more, and they are not mutually exclusive. In fact, they complement one another.

At the core, we crave purpose and integrity. We know our lives are not isolated events. We are connected to everything that preceded us and everything that will follow. If you have an overarching sense of direction, purpose, and connectedness, you will be more resilient, better able to manage the stressful events that could disrupt your equanimity and destroy your health. The restoration techniques we discuss in this chapter will ground you and center you as they relax you. Your goal is to experience peace, self-awareness, and thoughtful reflection. Most of us are preoccupied with living, thinking, organizing, and working. An appreciation of the wonder of everyday life will remove you from the chaotic pace that threatens to overwhelm you.

By now you have probably realized that **belief becomes biology.** Regardless of your stress type, connecting to a force greater than yourself will help bring relief. Your thoughts, feelings, and hopes produce and are produced by chemical and electrical activity in the nerve cells of your brain, and that affects your entire being. A belief in God, a higher power, a greater or deeper reality, or belonging to a community with shared beliefs diminishes the importance of your personal problems and worries, which seem insignificant in the greater scheme of things. The belief in something that transcends your individual existence can elevate you and remove you from day-to-day exigencies.

**While meditation is a monologue, prayer is a conversation.** Prayer is a conversation with a force greater than yourself. Prayer can take many forms. A prayer can be a thanksgiving, a plea for guidance or help, a confession, a request for forgiveness and redemption, praise, a profound commitment, worship, or surrender. Praying means that you have given up control, that you realize your power over the events in your life is limited. Acknowledging that you are not in charge of everything can be a freeing revelation. Prayer, a powerful way to reduce stress, can elevate you and comfort you in times of need and in your daily life.

## RELIGION, SPIRITUALITY, AND MEDICINE

Most studies show that religious involvement and spirituality are associated with better health, greater longevity, increased coping skills, better health-related quality of life, and less anxiety, depression, and suicide. Yet, medicine continues to ignore the spiritual needs of patients.

Belief is personal, but acknowledging and supporting a patient's spiritual needs does not have to be controversial. Spiritual beliefs and practices help to create a personally meaningful world. This reality is particularly important in the face of illness, disability, and death. We hope that in the future, medicine will incorporate the spiritual aspect of our lives into the system.

In our final chapter, "The Stress-Detox Program for Your Type," which follows, we will combine our recommendations in a program designed specifically for particular types of stress response.

CHAPTER NINE

# THE STRESS-DETOX PROGRAM
# FOR YOUR TYPE

Now that you are familiar with a wide range of options for reducing your physical and psychological stress, we want to put
it all together. We have recommendations for nutrition, exercise, and restoration techniques that we believe will provide the most
effective relief for particular stress types. Each type of stress response
has its own vulnerability. Though you cannot eliminate life's challenges and conflicts, there are many areas that you can control; our
suggestions are designed to help you do just that. They are not written
in stone and you should, of course, consult with your own physician
before implementing any of our suggestions.

Try not to be too ambitious at the start. You do not want to put
unreasonable demands on yourself and your time. If you do, it will become too easy for you to revert to your prior habits of inadequate nutrition, too little exercise, and no time to restore yourself. Instead, ease
into the program. After you have familiarized yourself with the strategic eating plan for your type, begin by making one change, whether
it is gradually cutting back on the amount of coffee you drink, eating
a healthy breakfast, or adding more fruits and vegetables to your diet.
Once you have mastered that first goal, move on to the next. If you
have not been exercising at all, start at the lowest intensity and duration for your type. The key is to be consistent and to build to thirty

minutes a day four or five times a week. Several of the restoration techniques take no more than fifteen to thirty minutes a day. It is essential that you set aside a total of a half hour a day to practice some form of stress management—and that time can be divided into a number of shorter time periods. We have included the time requirements for each type of exercise and technique in each program.

At the end of this chapter, we provide you with a Stress-Detox Program Log. You can reproduce it to keep track of how you are incorporating the elements of your Stress-Detox Program into your life. As you read through this chapter, you will see how little time your program actually demands of you. We hope you jump right into your program and enjoy the benefits of scientifically based stress relief.

## HyperS

Your program is designed to help you calm down. Your brain and nervous system are highly aroused. The best way for you to reduce your stress is to expend the energy that has been mobilized by your high cortisol level, so the most important element of the program for you is exercise. If you don't use that energy, it will be stored as fat. A regular, vigorous workout at the start of your day will provide the natural release of that mobilized energy and will defuse the tension you carry in your mind and body. You can make your workout a moving meditation, because your mind is also aroused and vigilant. Exercise will make your brain more resilient and less stress-sensitive.

We also want you to learn to relax your tense muscles. We recommend of number of relaxation techniques that will be most effective for you, especially progressive muscle relaxation. Consider doing progressive muscle relaxation in the evening to release tension that has built up during the day. If you follow the program described in the following pages, you will calm your body and mind.

# HyperS STRATEGIC NUTRITION PLAN

## AVOID COFFEE

You should consider giving up coffee for a number of reasons. Coffee is highly acidic and will promote extra cortisol production and arouse your already hyperaroused sympathetic nervous system; you are already high-strung enough without added caffeine jitters. If you cannot live without caffeine, try tea instead, green and white tea especially, because they have much less caffeine than coffee. The L-theanine in tea will give you the benefit of an alert mental state while it relaxes you. Tea is also more alkaline than coffee. If you simply cannot live without your coffee, wait until you have had the benefits of a good breakfast to have your first cup. Coffee alone not does not count as breakfast. To avoid withdrawal symptoms, taper off the caffeine slowly, by decreasing the amount of coffee you drink by four to six ounces every three days.

## ALKALINIZE YOUR pH

Acid alkaline balance is important for you. Since oxidative stress tends to be high for HyperSs, acidosis is a common condition for your type. Even mild acidosis can increase cortisol production, so your diet should be balanced by alkaline-producing foods at each meal. Check the chart on pages 155–56 for foods to incorporate into your meal and snack selections and those to avoid.

## BOOST TRYPTOPHAN AND TYROSINE

In order to calm your overstimulated nervous system and improve your mood, you need to consume foods that enable tryptophan to travel through the blood-brain barrier. Tryptophan is the building block for serotonin, the neurotransmitter that balances norepinephrine in your aroused brain. Boosting tryptophan levels will help maintain adequate serotonin levels to achieve this balance. You also need tyrosine to produce the norepinephrine your aroused brain is using. Tyrosine helps promote the production of norepinephrine in active neurons to protect them from burning out. A list of foods you should include in your diet appears on page 160.

## EAT LOW-GLYCEMIC FOODS

You need regular and steady glucose delivery to your brain, and you have to minimize your risks associated with insulin resistance, type 2 diabetes, central obesity, and heart disease. Foods that have a low glycemic index are right for you.

Aside from our short list of glycemic index in various foods on page 162, there are many online sources that will tell you how quickly various foods convert to sugars.

## GET THOSE ANTIOXIDANTS

Your wired nervous system is capable of producing a good deal of free-radical damage, so you need to counter this oxidative stress with antioxidants. As your stress type has a tendency to develop insulin resistance, eating antioxidant-rich foods is particularly important for you, because oxidative stress will further increase with insulin resistance. In addition to the antioxidant sources found on page 166, you should try drinking white tea, which has the highest antioxidant effects and is low in caffeine compared with other types of tea.

## SPECIAL MICRONUTRIENT NEEDS

HyperSs are often susceptible to colds, sinus infections, cold sores, and bladder infections. You need immune-boosting foods that contain vitamin C and zinc. Aside from your multivitamin, you should take 1000–3000 mg. of vitamin C a day and ten to thirty mg. of zinc. You will find some sources of vitamin C and zinc listed in the micronutritional section that begins on page 131.

## SKIP THE NIGHTCAP

We recommend that you limit the amount of alcohol you drink. Though it initially has a calming effect, more than five drinks per week is not a good idea. Drinking too much alcohol will dehydrate you and can disrupt your already problematic sleep.

## MEAL COMPOSITION AND TIMING

Breakfast should be your largest meal, because insulin resistance increases throughout the day, and you can consume more nutrients and calories in the morning with less tendency to gain weight. Pack your breakfast with nutritionally dense foods such as eggs, dairy, fruits, berries, and whole-grain breads. If you choose eggs for breakfast, scramble them with some alkalinizing spinach and tomatoes. Molasses, an alkaline rich in iron, is a great substitute for jam or jelly on your whole-grain bread.

We recommend that you have small meals at traditional lunch and dinner times and two small snacks, one in the late morning and one in the late afternoon. By eating a large meal in the morning and smaller meals the rest of the day, you will minimize the effects of a nervous stomach on your digestion. Even better, you will be less likely to gain weight. Calories consumed in the morning will be metabolized more efficiently than late in the day, when more insulin will be produced from the same caloric intake.

A good beverage choice for you is kombucha, a fermented tea that you can find refrigerated in the raw-foods section of many health stores. Kombucha has very little caffeine and is rich in probiotics, which have an immune-boosting effect. This fermented tea is alkaline and will help to keep your pH in balance. Do not drink too much kombucha; about four ounces should be enough to reap all the benefits. The bacterial flora stimulated by any probiotic can overgrow and cause bloating and vaginal irritation.

## HyperS EXERCISE PLAN

**Exercise is the most important part of the program for HyperSs.** Since you have a chronically mobilized fight-or-flight response, exercise is the natural antidote to your allostatic load. Regular daily exercise for thirty minutes will promote the production of serotonin, dopamine, endorphins, and neuropeptides, which are known to protect neurons involved in learning and memory. Not only will your mood be improved, but stress-induced damage to your brain will be prevented. This will make you less susceptible to future stress and will also protect your memory.

Our goals for you are:

- Energy utilization
- Reduction in weight gain around your middle
- Improved insulin sensitivity
- Better blood-lipid profiles; improved mood, memory, and sleep

Your high cortisol and insulin levels make mornings the perfect time to exercise regularly. Since you tend to wake up ready to go, with your mind full of things to do, jogging, cycling, or running can be a form of moving meditation for you. Try to break a sweat once a day.

**Aerobic exercise** of moderate to high intensity is appropriate, depending on your level of fitness. Anything that gets your heart pumping will do: walking briskly, jogging, using an elliptical machine or stationary bike, and taking aerobics classes are just a few of the ways you can get moving. If your morning schedule does not allow for more than a few minutes of exercise, we suggest jumping rope or running in place.

**Time:** thirty minutes a day, at least five times a week.

**Weight training** or other anaerobic, strength-training programs are appropriate for you. The rhythmic contractions of the large muscle groups stimulate the uptake of glucose into muscles and improve energy utilization and insulin resistance. The balance in your body is shifted toward energy oxidation instead of energy storage. This will help specifically with central weight gain, overall metabolism, cholesterol levels, and oxidative stress.

**Time:** fifteen to twenty minutes two or three times a week, not on sequential days.

Given the tendency of HyperSs to be apples, you might want to incorporate some **Pilates** into your exercise program. Pilates focuses on core strength and works your abdominal muscles. If you have a lot of pent-up energy, you might want to take up kickboxing or martial arts.

**Time:** fifteen to thirty minutes of Pilates mat work as often as you like.

## HyperS RESTORATION

Restoration for HyperSs will center on four key strategies:

- Quiet your overstimulated mind
- Relax overly tense muscles
- Achieve lower cortisol levels
- Restore balance between the parasympathetic nervous system and the sympathetic nervous system

The goal is to enhance your physiological and psychological adaptability. Experiment with different techniques to find one or a combination that works well for you. Our specific recommendations for your type are:

- Use the **ABCDE method** (see chapter 2) to deconstruct negative or self-defeating thought patterns and feelings.
  **Time:** ten to fifteen minutes.

- **Manage your time** by prioritizing and learning to say no. Do not let your to-do list overwhelm you.
  **Time:** five minutes.

- **Diaphragmatic breathing** can be helpful at night to prepare for sleep or anytime during the day that you feel your stress levels rising.
  **Time:** three to five minutes several times a day.

- **Mindfulness meditation** when you wake in the morning and before dinner. Since HyperSs tend to have very active "monkey minds," this practice will make you aware of the agitated thoughts that constantly race through your mind. Mindfulness meditation will distance you from the internal pressure you put on yourself.
  **Time:** work up to two sessions of twenty minutes twice a day, preferably before breakfast and dinner.

- **Progressive muscle relaxation** will help you relieve the characteristic tension that you, as a HyperS, carry in your body, particularly your facial muscles. If you want to avoid developing a furrowed brow, frown lines, or other wrinkles, learn to scan for tension in your face and to relax those muscles. This can be done in the evening to ease the day's tension.
  **Time:** five minutes three times a day.

- **Journaling** can provide an outlet for your anxieties and perseverations. If you set aside a specific time each day, you can write about what is troubling you. The ritual can cleanse your mind of your worries and keep you from obsessing about things. Keep a notebook next to your bed as well. If you wake

up at night with your mind full of disruptive ruminations, write them down. Organizing your thoughts to put them down in writing can make them less disturbing.
**Time:** ten to fifteen minutes.

- **Deep tissue massage** will rid your body of knots of tension. Touch can stimulate oxytocin production and the ensuing cascade of feel-good neurotransmitters.
**Time:** twenty to thirty minutes.

- **Aromatherapy and reflexology** will be very soothing. A foot massage using lavender oil prior to going to bed will also stimulate the oxytocin pathway. Lavender enhances the parasympathetic nervous system, which will balance out your hyperactive sympathetic nervous system. Lavender also increases the scavenging of reactive oxygen free-radial species (ROS), reducing oxidative stress.
**Time:** ten to thirty minutes.

- **Tai chi** can be beneficial for your type because the martial arts movements will help you to control your energy.
**Time:** twenty to forty minutes.

- **Prayer** or recognizing a higher power will reenforce that you are not responsible for everything, that many things are beyond your control.
**Timeless.**

## HypoS

A triad of symptoms is associated with your stress type: fatigue, pain, and stress sensitivity. Our program for you is designed to entrain and enhance your cortisol levels. This will balance your unchecked sympathetic nervous system, make you more resilient and less sensitive to stress, and calm your overzealous immune system.

**Nutrition and restoration are equally important parts of your program.** The nutritional strategies in the program will show you how to correct your blunted cortisol release by the timing of your meals and what you eat. The restoration will strengthen the brain pathways that modulate your intense stress response.

One of cortisol's many roles is to keep your immune system in check. Since your cortisol levels are low when you are stressed, your immune system becomes overactive, which leads to inflammation, pain, and disease. Eating anti-inflammatory foods, especially omega-3s, and paying close attention to your vitamin-D level will help to curb the aggressive behavior of your immune system. Calcium, folate, and B12 are important for you as well.

Your major vulnerability is your extreme sensitivity to stress. You can control your overly excitable stress response by anticipating and managing potentially stressful situations. Living in an organized and structured way can eliminate a good deal of stress from your life. Restoration techniques that promote balance between your parasympathetic and sympathetic nervous systems will make you more adaptable and stress-resistant. Over time, our program for you will revitalize you and restore your joie de vivre.

## HypoS STRATEGIC NUTRITION PLAN

### STIMULATE ENDORPHIN PRODUCTION

Since HypoSs often struggle with chronic pain, you will want to stimulate your brain to produce more endorphins. The foods that are most effective in boosting endorphin production are those that are sweet and creamy; eating a small piece of dark chocolate (70 percent cocoa) can actually give you some pain relief.

## CONSUME MORE TYROSINE- AND TRYPTOPHAN-CONTAINING FOODS

Since your sympathetic nervous system and brain are easily activated, your body needs tyrosine and tryptophan to produce serotonin and dopamine, neurotransmitters that can balance you. This is a good reason to have protein at each meal, but remember to include complex carbohydrates in your meal so that tryptophan can pass through the blood-brain barrier. You can find a list of the sources of tyrosine and tryptophan on pages 157–59.

## EAT FOODS WITH LOW GLYCEMIC INDEX

Your activated sympathetic nervous system promotes insulin resistance. Even though your cortisol level is not elevated, as it is with a HyperS, your nervous system is very aroused and needs the constant, steady energy that this type of diet provides. You do not tolerate reactive hypoglycemia. Making sure that you avoid foods with a high glycemic index will help to lower your risk of insulin resistance and such diseases as type 2 diabetes, heart disease, and obesity, which might develop. You can find a list of the glycemic index of a number of foods on page 162. If you want a more extensive list and one that features brands, check the internet, where many comprehensive lists are available.

## DON'T FORGET THE ANTIOXIDANTS

Your overactive nervous system and immune system can create free-radical damage. You will need antioxidants to counter this oxidative stress. Since HypoSs tend to develop insulin resistance, you will need to consume foods rich in antioxidants, because they have insulin-sensitizing effects. A list of antioxidant-packed foods appears on pages 166–67.

## ANTI-INFLAMMATORY FOODS ARE PARTICULARLY IMPORTANT

Your immune system tends to work overtime and can damage your organs. Women who have a HypoS stress response have a tendency to develop allergies, asthma, and irritable bowel function. You can help to combat this proclivity with anti-inflammatory foods. These are foods rich in omega-3 fatty acids, such as fish, olive oil, and walnuts. Consider free-range eggs for breakfast with whole-grain toast for a good source of omega-3s in the morning.

## SPECIAL MICRONUTRIENT NEEDS

You should take a multivitamin containing all the supplements listed in the micronutritional insurance section that begins on page 131. You should also consider supplementing your diet with vitamin D3 (dosage depends on sun exposure) for its autoimmune-disease-preventing action. HypoSs with inflammatory bowel issues may have a special need for fat-soluble vitamins A (700 IU to a maximum of 300 IU) and E (15–1000 mg.) because you may not be absorbing these nutrients from your food.

## MEAL COMPOSITION AND TIMING

The timing of your meals is very important because your cortisol rhythm is blunted. You can help to entrain your cortisol rhythm by establishing a routine of eating each meal at the same time every day. You should eat near traditional mealtimes, but it is important to establish a schedule that works for you. A diet high in fiber from fruits and vegetables is particularly important for your type. This will help to maintain proper bacterial function of your sensitive bowels and meet your need for foods low in glycemic index. Raw cabbage and raw beets are especially good for this. Pay careful attention to staying well hydrated as well to help your sensitive digestive tract.

Since morning energy can be a problem for you, a small cup of coffee now and then is fine to jump-start your body. You should use coffee only occasionally, when you need an added boost to get going. Your activated sympathetic nervous system does not need the extra stimulation that coffee provides every day. Instead, you should drink white and green teas, which contain less caffeine, are alkaline, and create calm arousal (see pages 155–56).

Eating lunch is associated with the largest boost in cortisol during the day. Since cortisol production needs to be stimulated for HypoSs, eating your main meal at midday will augment that rise in cortisol. If you eat a lunch that is carbohydrate heavy, you run the risk of crashing soon after you finish. We recommend a meal that is high in protein and complex carbohydrates. An ideal lunch for you would be a salad of mixed greens and arugla with a citrus vinaigrette, grilled fish or chicken, and vegetables. This combination of foods is perfect for your type. It provides the amino acids, essential fatty acids, and antioxidants you need. Breakfast and dinner should be smaller meals than lunch, but nutrient balance is important throughout the day. Snacks are not essential for your type if your meal schedule is regular.

## HypoS EXERCISE

Exercise will help with your aches and pains and lessen the stress sensitivity of your brain. Though you might feel too tired and have little to no energy, exercise will dramatically improve your vitality and reduce your pain. It can be hard for you to get going in the morning, but exercising at the same time every day will help to entrain your biological rhythms. We advise exercising in natural daylight when possible or at least near a window with natural light.

We do not expect you to train for a marathon or take up boxing. What is most important is for you to be consistent. Start slowly and build intensity after you are able to maintain thirty minutes of exercise at least three days a week. You have to start slowly and gradually increase the length of time you exercise and the intensity of your workouts. Once you get moving, you will feel so much better that you will look forward to the time you schedule for exercise. Our goals include:

- Entraining biorhythms
- Reducing pain and boosting energy
- Raising energy levels
- Improving mood and making the brain less sensitive to stress
- Stimulating the oxytocin pathways

## REDUCING PAIN AND BOOSTING ENERGY

Rhythmic, gentle, low-impact movements are appropriate for HypoSs. Stretching should be part of your daily routine, since keeping your body supple will relieve muscle pain. You might enjoy riding a bike, taking a water aerobics class, ballroom dancing, or hatha yoga. The fact is that the more energy you expend, the more energy you have, providing that you do not overdo it. The major stumbling block is just to get started. Once you do, you will feel like a different person; you will forget how sluggish you felt when you were a couch potato. Remember, those of you who are physically and psychologically less fit when you start will enjoy the quickest results and the most benefit from exercise.

## IMPROVING MOOD AND MEMORY

Regular aerobic activity will stimulate the production of endorphins, serotonin, and dopamine, which will make you feel better. Although your cortisol levels are lower than those of HyperSs, you still have an overly aroused sympathetic nervous system that requires management. Routine exercise will protect you from repeated hyperactivity of your sympathetic nervous system and prevent or reverse the damage to memory and mood that occurs with chronic stress.

## TEND-AND-BEFRIEND

Since socialization is so important for women in preventing or managing allostatic load, you would benefit from a regular walking routine with a friend. If your fitness level allows, you might want to take a Pilates or low-impact-aerobics class with a group of friends.

## HypoS RESTORATION

Restoration for HypoSs will center on four key strategies:

- Reduce or eliminate chronic pain
- Raise energy levels
- Improve immune function
- Enhance parasympathetic response and strengthen the vagal break

Our goal for your type is to help you deal with symptoms that can be debilitating. You can choose a technique that appeals to you from the list that follows. Once you have mastered one, try another. Our specific recommendations include:

- Using **cognitive therapy** and the **ABCDE model** to recognize negative thought patterns.
  **Time:** ten to fifteen minutes.

- **Diaphragmatic breathing** can be done multiple times during the day. Deep breathing can give you calming energy.
  **Time:** three minutes several times a day.

- **Aromatherapy** can be very soothing. Lavender will increase parasympathetic activity and rosemary has immune benefits.
  **Time:** fifteen to thirty minutes.

- **Mantra meditation** and emptying your mind should relieve you of draining thoughts and provide you with fresh energy.
  **Time:** build to twenty minutes before breakfast and twenty minutes before dinner.

- The warmth and heaviness employed in **autogenic training** can ease the pain of aching muscles.
  **Time:** ten to forty minutes twice a day.

- **Shiatsu massage and reflexology** deal with pressure points and energy flow in your body and can help you achieve a full-body release.
  **Time:** twenty to thirty minutes.

- **Biofeedback** can be very helpful for your type, because you need to control your sympathetic nervous system. You will have to focus on heart-rate variability to improve your vagal brake.
  **Time:** twenty minutes.

- **Qigong** can help you to center yourself and calm your mind.
  **Time:** twenty minutes.

- **Prayer** will take you outside yourself and help you to transcend pain and fatigue.
  **Timeless.**

## HypoP

Your extreme stress response makes it very difficult for you to make changes in your life. When you are stressed, you become severely overwhelmed and withdrawn, but with incremental changes you can reengage with the world. Our program for you is designed to enhance your mind-body connection, to improve your perception of yourself, and to bring you back to your life.

The most important part of the program for you is restoration. Keeping a journal will help you connect to your feelings, both physical and emotional. If you are unable to express your feelings, your stress will only intensify, transforming you into an observer of your life. Your goal is to heighten your engagement in the world and to generate a sense of control.

Though your profound exhaustion may prevent you from exercising, we suggest that you commit to short periods of physical activity each day. As you start, your tolerance for physical activity will be very low, but don't be discouraged. Just move your body in very small ways. Try walking outside for five minutes a day. Being out in the world and in natural light will help you to reconnect. Your biorhythms are severely out of sync. Meal timing, light exposure, and physical activity will help to lift and entrain your dampened systems and to bring your body into balance.

## HypoP STRATEGIC NUTRITION PLAN

### EASILY DIGESTIBLE FOODS

Many HypoPs have inflammatory bowel issues, which should be taken into account when selecting food. The foods you eat should be good for digestive function. We recommend eating high-fiber foods that do not create bloating, such as fruits and whole grains; raw vegetables and dairy can cause gastrointestinal problems for you, so consider cooked vegetables and sheep's milk or sheep's yogurt as alternatives. Probiotics will help to promote optimal bowel function. Drinking kombucha, a fermented tea, will provide cultures of healthy bacteria to promote the optimal gastrointestinal environment. Just remember, do not drink more than four ounces at a time.

## ANTI-INFLAMMATORY FOODS

Your low cortisol production and overactive immune system increase your need for anti-inflammatory foods. Foods rich in omega-3s, such as olive oil, salmon, and walnuts, will help calm inflammation. Check page 164 for a fuller list of foods rich in omega-3. Foods containing antioxidants, listed on pages 166–67, are also anti-inflammatory. Pineapple slices are anti-inflammatory and would make a good snack.

## SPECIAL MICRONUTRIENT NEEDS

You should consider taking a multivitamin with all the supplements listed in the Micronutritional Insurance section that begins on page 131. Vitamin D3 (dose, dependent on sun exposure), is particularly important for you to help prevent ulcerative colitis and Crohn's disease. You should take the fat-soluble vitamins, including A (700 IU to a maximum of 3000 IU) and E (15–1000 mg.), because you may not be absorbing these nutrients from your food.

## MEAL COMPOSITION AND TIMING

Since HypoPs have a blunted cortisol curve throughout the day, you need to synchronize your circadian rhythm by having specific mealtimes. We suggest that you have meals at traditional times. Lunch should be your largest meal, to boost cortisol release at that time. It should contain protein and complex carbohydrates. A sandwich made with turkey on whole-grain bread and a side of fruit is a good lunch for you. Skipping meals is not a good idea, as your body already struggles with dyssynchronized rhythms. Entrainment is very important for HypoPs to promote healthy sleep patterns, body temperature, blood pressure, hormone production, digestion, and immune activity. You do not have to be too concerned about glycemic index or load because your dominant parasympathetic system is insulin-sensitizing. That does not mean that you should eat processed foods made from white flour and sugar, because they contain very little nutrition. You should focus on carbohydrates that come from whole-food sources, such as whole grains, fruits, and berries. Your shut-down system needs nutritional support. You may need more carbohydrates than the other types to promote energy.

A whole-grain cereal, oatmeal or a grain mixture, is a good choice for breakfast. Avoid instant or quick varieties of oatmeal, which have been robbed of nutrients, and breakfast cereals that contain preservatives and sweeteners. You can drink coffee as long as you do not develop intestinal cramps. Green or white tea would be a better choice because of its alkaline and antioxidant properties.

## HypoP EXERCISE

Exercise for HypoPs should be started at a very low level and preferably in natural sunlight. It is important for you to exercise at the same time each day to entrain your biological rhythms so that your cortisol production becomes regulated to synchronize your system.

Our exercise goals for HypoPs are:

- Entrain biological rhythms
- Help to engage and participate in the world around them
- Improve strength, endurance, and flexibility over a gradual time frame

Since HypoPs tend to have low energy, you have to ease into exercise. Don't expect to run five miles on a treadmill or do the StairMaster for twenty minutes. You can start by taking a five-minute walk each day and increasing the time you spend moving in the world, enjoying nature and the comings and goings of the people around you. Routine exercise in natural daylight will help entrain your biorhythms. There are many wonderful exercise programs available on DVDs that have twenty-minute a.m. and p.m. stretching sequences; you can work out your arms with two-pound weights as you watch TV. There are so many enjoyable things you can do to move more, even window-shopping from one end of the mall to the other. Do not push yourself too hard; slowly and steadily is the way to go for you. In a matter of weeks, exercise will become a habit. You will find that you have more energy and a more optimistic point of view.

## HypoP RESTORATION

**Restoration is a priority for you.** Since HypoPs have severely imbalanced hormonal, immune, and neurological pathways, our recommendations for restoration techniques are directed to improving your mind-body communication. Being more in touch with your body will carry over to how you respond and function in the world.

Following is a list of restoration techniques that work well for your type. Simply choose one that appeals to you and experiment with others when you are ready. Our specific recommendations include:

**ABCDE method** (see chapter 2) of deconstructing your automatic reactions and faulty thinking that lead to negative emotions could help you to understand that your perception of events can be distorted.
**Time:** fifteen to thirty minutes.

**Diaphragmatic breathing** can be done multiple times during the day. It will give you calming energy.
**Time:** five minutes three times a day.

**Journaling** is very important for you. Recording what you experience each day will make you aware of how your thoughts, feelings, and body are interconnected.
**Time:** forty-five minutes every day.

**Autogenic training** will increase the activity of your sympathetic nervous system, and the warmth and heaviness you create will be comforting.
**Time:** ten to forty minutes twice a day.

**Aromatherapy** with lavender or rosemary will enhance your immune system and soothe your weariness.
**Time:** fifteen to thirty minutes.

**Shiatsu massage** will help to balance your disrupted, desynchronized system by focusing on acupressure meridian points in your body.
**Time:** twenty minutes.

**Swedish massage** will help to improve the circulation to your aching muscles and joints.
**Time:** thirty to fifty minutes.

**Biofeedback** can be very helpful for you. Learning to identify the cues your body sends you will help you to balance your autonomic nervous system, improving your sympathetic tone. Learning biofeedback can give you a sense of control over your body, which you need in order to handle your extreme stress response.
**Time:** twenty to forty-five minutes.

**Prayer** will connect you to a power greater than yourself, taking you outside yourself and giving you a sense of your place in the universe.
**Timeless.**

# HyperP

Your program is twofold. You have to learn how to prevent your collapses as well as how to restore yourself when you have had a meltdown. For someone so accomplished at multitasking, your periodic collapses and inability to function are a very urgent message from your body. You are so focused on balancing all the things in your life that you have lost touch with what the stress of your very full life is doing to your mind and body.

No matter how other women appear on the outside, be assured that there are no wonder women in the real world. Revising your notions of what you should do and accomplish and prioritizing in a self-protective way will relieve your stress. The preventive part of your program involves time management. You have to resist overcommitting your time and energy. Learn to say no, and try not make everything on your to-do list a top priority.

When stress has wiped you out, you will recover more quickly if you pamper yourself. Soothing music, a luxurious bath with scented oils, or reflexology or a massage will restore you. When you are in a completely drained state, you should refrain from exercising for a day or two to allow your body to unwind. You will need that time to bring your body back to balance. Building in time to restore yourself every day—even if it is only for twenty minutes—is essential for you. This small time investment each day will prevent you from being immobilized for a day or two. You need vigorous exercise to help you balance the energy mobilized by your precollapse stress response. Since you are susceptible to colds and flu, especially during wipeouts, your diet has to include immune-boosting nutrition and supplements.

# HyperP STRATEGIC NUTRITION PLAN

## TYROSINE LOADING

You have a tendency to crash because your norepinephrine becomes depleted. You need to load your diet with many sources of tyrosine. You can find a list on pages 157–59. We recommend that you start your day with eggs and yogurt. Most alcoholic beverages contain tyrosine, so if you are relaxing in the evening, consider having a small glass of something. Tyrosine is found in ale, beer, wine (especially port and Chianti), vermouth, and distilled spirits.

## IMMUNITY BUILDING

Your immune system is compromised by your high cortisol levels. In your transient state of collapse, you energy is so low that you are likely to get sick. In addition to taking a multivitamin, make sure your food has good sources of vitamin C and zinc to help build your immune response. You will need antioxidants for this purpose as well. You will find a list of food sources of these vitamins and mineral in the Micronutritional Insurance section, beginning on page 131.

## MEAL COMPOSITION AND TIMING

A small cup of coffee in the morning will give you energy and make you more alert. It may aggravate your sensitive stomach, which occurs from your dominant parasympathetic nervous system during this period. Do not drink coffee after noon because it is likely to disrupt your sleep, which you need to restore yourself.

Your meals should be simple because you need time to rest and get your energy back. Rather than have three big meals a day, eat small meals and snacks throughout the day when you are hungry to keep your energy level steady. Granola with nuts, slightly sweetened with sugar or honey, would be a good snack for you, and you could even consider a scoop of real ice cream for dessert for energy promotion and soothing effects.

# HyperP EXERCISE

Since HyperPs are in a temporary state of brain and body exhaustion that requires replenishing the norepinephrine levels in the brain, we advise that you refrain from exercising for at least one or two days as you recover from this state of depletion. The last thing you want to do is to push yourself: that is how you ended up in this condition. A leisurely walk in the sunshine or a casual bike ride should be enough. You might consider doing some gentle stretching exercises or hatha-yoga positions. Adding joyful music during gentle exercise will have a beneficial effect on your depleted brain.

When you are not in a state of collapse, you should exercise as a HyperS does. You need to exercise regularly to avoid the exhaustion that leads to your collapse.

# HyperP RESTORATION

The restoration guidelines for this passing state of depletion focus on restoring energy, balance, and vitality. Though your energy is practically nonexistent, the restoration techniques we suggest should be a pleasure. Our specific recommendations for your type are:

- **Diaphragmatic breathing** on awakening will help you begin the day with autonomic balance.
  **Time:** three minutes several times a day as you recuperate.

- **Swedish massage** will be stimulating and get your blood flowing again.
  **Time:** thirty to fifty minutes.

- **Tai chi** has controlled movements that could help to reenergize your body.
  **Time:** twenty minutes.

- **Pamper yourself**—try a day at a spa or an at-home spa day, a mani/pedi, or a small shopping spree. You need a day to focus on yourself for revitalization.
  **Time:** at least twenty minutes a day before you crash and a full day after you have crashed.

- **Prayer** can lift your spirits and bring light back into your life.
  **Timeless.**

The following pages provide you with a chart for each of the four Stress Detox Programs so that you can see our recommendations for your type in a glance.

## HyperS Program

### STRATEGIC NUTRITION

- Avoid caffeine
- Largest meal at breakfast
- Alkalinize your pH
- Boost tryptophan and tyrosine
- Low-glycemic-index foods
- Antioxidant-rich foods
- Immune-boosting nutrients, vitamin C, zinc
- Probiotics, best found in whole foods, not supplements
- Minimize alcohol consumption

### EXERCISE

- Exercise in the morning
- At least thirty minutes a day
- Try to break a sweat once a day
- Moderate- to high-intensity aerobics
- Weight training
- Pilates

### RESTORATION TECHNIQUES

- ABCDE method
- Time log
- Diaphragmatic breathing
- Mindful meditation
- Progressive muscle relaxation
- Journaling
- Deep-tissue massage
- Aromatherapy
- Tai chi
- Prayer

## HypoS

### STRATEGIC NUTRITION

- A balanced protein and complex-carbohydrate lunch for main meal
- Eat meals at the same time every day
- Eat foods that promote endorphin production
- Consume more tyrosine- and tryptophan-containing foods
- Low-glycemic index foods
- Antioxidants
- Anti-inflammatory foods
- Need vitamins D3, A, and E

### EXERCISE

- Work out at the same time every day
- Try to exercise in natural daylight or near a window
- Start slowly and build up
- Stretching
- Rhythmic, gentle, low-impact exercise is best
- Walk with a friend or pet
- Bike riding
- Water aerobics
- Hatha yoga
- Ballroom dancing
- Pilates
- Tai chi

### RESTORATION

- Cognitive therapy
- ABCDE model
- Diaphragmatic breathing
- Aromatherapy
- Mantra meditation
- Autogenic training
- Shiatsu massage
- Reflexology
- Prayer
- Yoga

## HypoP

### STRATEGIC NUTRITION

- Caffeine in morning
- Largest meal at lunch
- Meals at the same time every day
- Easily digestible foods—avoid raw vegetables and dairy
- Glycemic index less important
- Probiotics

### EXERCISE

- Same time each day
- Begin with five-minute walk each day to begin and increase gradually
- Gentle stretching

### RESTORATION

- ABCDE method
- Diaphragmatic breathing
- Journaling
- Mantra meditation
- Autogenic training
- Aromatherapy
- Biofeedback
- Shiatsu massage
- Swedish massage
- Prayer
- Yoga

## HyperP

### STRATEGIC NUTRITION

- Caffeine in the morning
- No caffeine in the afternoon
- Small meals and snacks during the day
- Tyrosine loading
- Antioxidants

### EXERCISE

- Leisurely walk
- Casual bike ride
- Gentle stretching
- Hatha yoga
- Music with exercise

### RESTORATION

- Diaphragmatic breathing
- Swedish massage
- Tai chi
- Pamper yourself
- Prayer

We have prepared a log page so that you can keep track of your efforts to change your life and return to balance, calm, and joy. Make copies of this page and keep it where you will see it to remind you of your commitment, to encourage you, and to measure the benefits of following your Stress-Detox Program.

**The Stress-Detox Program Log**

| Time of Day | Food Consumed | Vegetables and Fruit Consumed | Comments/Feelings |
|---|---|---|---|
|  |  |  |  |
|  |  |  |  |
|  |  |  |  |
|  |  |  |  |
|  |  |  |  |
|  |  |  |  |
|  |  |  |  |
|  |  |  |  |
|  |  |  |  |

Water ○○○○○○○○
Put a line through each circle for each eight-ounce glass

| Time of Day | Physical Activity | Duration/Intensity | Comments/Feelings Before and After |
|---|---|---|---|
|  |  |  |  |
|  |  |  |  |
|  |  |  |  |
|  |  |  |  |
|  |  |  |  |

| Time of Day | Restoration | Duration | Comments/Feelings Before and After |
|---|---|---|---|
|  |  |  |  |
|  |  |  |  |
|  |  |  |  |
|  |  |  |  |
|  |  |  |  |

# AFTERWORD

We hope that *The Ultimate Stress-Relief Plan for Women* has inspired you to make changes in the way you live to reduce the stress that we see plaguing our patients, friends, and families. You have the capacity to manage your reaction to stressful circumstances, to become more resilient, and to make your body stress-resistant. We have not given you simplistic solutions, which do not work in the long term. We have, to the best of our knowledge, given you the most-effective recommendations for your stress type, based on our clinical experience and the most recent science available, and a flexible program that is not unrealistically demanding, one that you can incorporate in your day-to-day life. Remember, it is human nature to fall back on old habits when you are under a lot of stress, but we want you also to remember that in stressful times you need to protect yourself the most. Be sensitive to when you begin to lean in that direction, and do your best to correct your mind-set and behavior. If you fall off your stress plan for whatever reason, just pick up where you left off.

We look forward to hearing from you about how your Stress-Detox Program has affected you. We hope you will communicate with us at our website www.sostressedonline.com. Just as our patients have helped us with this book, we are eager for you to share with us what works for you to relieve stress. We plan to offer even more information, tips, and inspiration on our site to encourage you to do everything you can to restore your balance, energy, and joy.

Motivated by what we see in our practice every day and what we have learned about dealing with stress, we are in the process of extending the work we have begun in *The Ultimate Stress-Relief Plan for Women* by establishing a center for stress management, an expansion of our current practice.

What we want most is for you to finish this book with a spirit of hope and confidence. We want you to be committed to adopting the nutritional, exercise, and restoration techniques we have suggested and to embrace the control you have over your response to stress.

# SELECTED BIBLIOGRAPHY

Since this is not an academic book, we have not provided footnotes for each chapter. Instead, we have listed the sources we found most valuable to us in our research.

## Chapter 2: The Psychology of Stress

Aspinwell, L. G., and S. E. Taylor. "A Stitch in Time: Self-Regulation and Proactive Coping." *Psychological Bulletin* 121 (1997): 417–36.

Bergeron, Louis. "Suppression As a Coping Mechanism Increased Stress," *Stamford News Service*. March 24, 2008.

Brennan, Penny L., Kathleen K. Schutte, and Rudolf H. Moos. "Long Term Patterns and Predictors of Successful Stressor Resolution in Later Life." *International Journal of Stress Management* 13, no. 3 (2006): 253–72.

Burns, David D., MD. *The Feeling Good Handbook*. New York: William Morrow, 1989.

Degangi, Georgie A., Stephen W. Porges, Ruth Z. Sickel, and Stanley I. Greenspan. "Four-Year Follow Up of a Sample of Regulatory Disordered Infants." *Infant Mental Health Journal* 14, no. 4 (February 2006): 330–43.

Doussard-Roosevelt, Jane A., Bonita D. McClenny, and Stephen W. Porges. "Neonatal Cardio-Vagal Tone and School Age Development Outcomes in Very Low Birth Weight Infants." *Developmental Psychobiology* 38, issue 1 (2001): 56–66.

Doussard-Roosevelt, Jane A., Stephen W. Porges, John W. Scanlon, Behjat

Alemi, and Kathleen B. Scanlon. "Vagal Regulation of Heart Rate in the Prediction of Developmental Outcome for Very Low Birth Weight Preterm Infants." *Child Development* 68, issue 2 (2008): 173–87.

Ellis, Albert. *Overcoming Destructive Beliefs, Feelings, and Behaviors.* Amherst, New York: Prometheus Books, 2001.

Ellis, Albert, PhD, and Catherine MacLauren, MSW. *Rational Emotive Behavior Therapy: A Therapist's Guide.* San Luis Obispo, CA: Impact Publishers, 1998.

Ellis, Albert, PhD, and Robert A. Hamper, PhD. *A New Guide for Rational Living.* North Hollywood, CA: Wilshire, 1975.

Emery, Gary, PhD. *Getting Undepressed: How a Woman Can Change Her Life through Cognitive Therapy,* revised edition. New York: Touchstone, 1988.

Emotional Analysis—Stress Management Techcniques from MindTools, www.mindtools.com/stress/rt/EmotionalAnalysis.htm.

Folkman, Susan, and Judith Moskowitz. "Stress, Positive Emotion, and Coping." *Current Directions in Psychological Science* 9, issue 4 (August 2000): 115.

Goldberger, Leo, and Shlomo Bretznitz. *The Handbook of Stress: Theoretical and Clinical Aspects,* second edition. New York: Free Press, 1992.

Goleman, Daniel. *Emotional Intelligence.* New York: Bantam Books, 1995.

Greenberger, Dennis, and Christine A. Padesky. *Mind over Mood: Change How You Feel by Changing the Way You Think.* New York: Guilford Press, 1995.

Hammerfeld, K. C. Ebele, M. Grau, A. Kinsperga, A. Zimmerman, V. Ehlert, and J. Gaab. "Persistent Effects of Cognitive-Behavioral Stress Management of Cortisol Responses to Acute Stress in Healthy Subjects—A Randomized Controlled Trial." *Psychoendocrinology* 31, issue 3 (April 2006): 333–39.

Kiuimaki, Mika, Marko Elouainio, Archana Singh-Maroux, Tussi Vahlera, Hans Helenius, and Jaana Pentij. "Optimism/Pessimism as Predictors of Change in Health after Death or Onset of Severe Illness in Family." *Health Psychology* 24, no. 4 (2005): 413–21.

Kosaka, Moritaka, "Relationship between Hardiness and Psychological Stress Response." *Journal of Performance Studies* 3 (1996): 35–40.

Lazarus, Richard S. "Why We Should Think of Stress As a Subset of Emotion." *The Handbook of Stress,* eds. Leo Goldenberger and Shlomo Breznitz. New York: Free Press, 1993.

———. *Stress and Emotion: A New Synthesis.* New York: Springer Publishing, 1999.

———, and Bernice N. Lazarus. *Passion and Reason: Making Sense of Our Emotions.* New York: Oxford University Press, 1954.

———, and Susan Folkman. *Stress Appraisal and Coping.* New York: Springer Publishing, 1984.

Monat, Alan, and Richard S. Lazarus. *Stress and Coping: An Anthology,* third edition. New York: Columbia University Press, 1991.

Peterson, Christopher, Martin E. Seligman, and George E. Vaillant. "Harvard Study on Pessimism." *Journal of Personality and Social Psychology* 55, no. 1 (1988): 23–27.

Rafnsson, Fjolvar Darri, Fridrik H. Jonsson, and Michael Windle. "Coping Strategies, Stressful Life Events, Problem Behaviors, and Depressed Affect." *Anxiety, Stress, and Coping* 19, issue 3 (September 2006): 241–57.

Veron, E., T. E. Joier, F. Johnson, and T. Benter. "Gender Specific Gene Environment Interactions on Laboratory Assessed Aggression." *Biological Psychology* 71: 33–41.

## Chapter 3: The Anatomy of Stress and Chapter 4:
### Identify Your Stress Type

Adolphus, Ralph. "Social Cognition and the Human Brain." In *Foundations in Social Neuroscience,* eds. John T. Cacioppo, Gary G.

Berntson, Ralph Adolphus, et al. Cambridge, MA: Bradford Books, MIT Press, 2002: 313–32.

Alexander, Joanne Levanthal, Lorraine Dennerstein, Nancy Fugate Woods, Bruce S. McEwen, Uriel Halbreich, Krista Kotz, and Gregg Richardson. "The Role of Stressful Events and Menopausal Stage in Well-Being and Health." *Expert Rev. Neurotherapeutics* 7, no. 11 (2007): S93–S113.

Andeano, Joseph M., and Larry Cahill. "Sex Differences in the Neurobiology of Learning and Memory. *Learning and Memory,* (2009).

Arrone, Louis J., MD, and Alisa Bowman. *The Skinny: On Losing Weight without Being Hungry—the Ultimate Guide to Weight Loss Success.* New York: Broadway Books, 2009.

Baker, Roger A., Stephen Barasi, with Neuropharmacology by M.J. Neal. *Neuroscience at a Glance,* third edition. Malden, MA: Blackwell, 2008.

Bakewell, Dr. S. "The Autonomic Nervous System." http://www.think body.co.uk/papers/autonomic-nervous-system.htm.

Bear, Mark F., Barry W. Cannos, and Michael A. Paradiso. *Neuroscience: Exploring the Brain,* third edition. Baltimore: Lippincott, Williams, and Wilkins, 2007.

Becker, Jill B., Arthur P. Arnold, Karen J. Berkley, Jeffrey D. Blaustein, Lisa A. Eckel, Elizabeth Hampson, James P. Herna, Sherry Marts, Wolfgang Sadea, Meir Steiner, June Taylor, and Elizabeth Young. *Endocrinology* 146 (4): 1650–73.

Becto-Fernandez, Luis, Teresa Rodriguez-Cano, Esther Delayo-Delgado, and Myralys Calaf. "Are There Gender-Specific Pathways from Early Adolescence Psychological Distress Symptoms Toward the Development of Substance Use and Abnormal Eating Behavior?" *Child Psychiatry and Human Development* 37 (2007): 193–203.

Beer, Jennifer S. "The Importance of Emotion-Social Cognition Interactions for Social Functioning: Insights from Orbitofrontal

Cortex." *Social Neuroscience: Integrating Biological and Psychological Explanations of Social Behavior.* Eddi Harmon-Jones and Piotr Winkielman. New York: The Guilford Press, 2007.

Bjoprntop, Per, and Roland Rosmond. "The Metabolic Syndrome—a Neuroendocrine Disorder?" *British Journal of Nutrition* 83, Suppl. 1 (2000): S49–S47.

———. "Obesity and Cortisol." *Nutrition* 16, no. 10 (2000): 924–36.

*Britannica Guide to the Brain: A Guided Tour of the Brain, Mind, Memory, and Intelligence.* London: Constable and Robinson, 2008.

Cahill, Larry. "His Brain, Her Brain." In *Scientific American* 292, no. 5 (May 2005), 40–47.

———. "Why Sex Matters for Neuroscience." *Nature Reviews Neuroscience,* 7477–84, June 2006.

Carter, C. S., B. Kirkpatrick, and I. I. Lederlender. (eds). *The Integrative Neurobiology of Affliation.* Cambridge, MA: MIT Press, 1999.

Carter, C. Sue. "Neuropeptides and the Protective Effects of Social Bonds." In *Social Neuroscience,* Eddie Harmon-Jones and Piotr Winkielman, eds. New York: Guilford Press, 2007: 425–38.

Charmandari, Evangelia, Constantine Tsigos, and George P. Chrousos. "Endocrinology of the Stress Response." *Annual Review Physiology* 67 (2005): 259–84.

———, Tomoshige Kino, and George P. Chrousos. "Glucocorticoids and Their Actions: An Introduction." *Annals of the New York Academy of Science* 1024 1-8 (2004).

Charney, Dennis S., MD. "Psychobiological Mechanisms of Resilience and Vulnerability: Implications for Successful Adaptation to Extreme Stress. *Focus* 11, no. 3 (summer 2004): 368–91.

Chrousos, George P., and Philip W. Gold. "The Concepts of Stress and Stress System Disorders." *JAMA* 267, no. 9 (March 4, 1992): 1244–51.

———, David J. Torpy, and Philip W. Gold. "Interaction Between HPA Axis and Female Reproductive System" *Annals of Internal Medicine* 129, no. 3 (August 1998): 229–40.

Cohen, Sheldon, Ellen Frank, William J. Doyle, David P. Skover, Bruce S. Rabin, and Jack M. Gwaltney Jr. "Types of Stresses That Increase Susceptibility to the Common Cold in Healthy Adults." In *Foundations of Social Neuroscience* op. cit.: 1229–40.

———, Ronald Kessler, and Lynn Underwood Gordon. *Measuring Stress: A Guide for Health and Social Scientists.* New York: Oxford University Press, 1995.

———, David Tyrell, and Andrew P. Smith. "Psychological Stress and Susceptibility to the Common Cold." In *Psychosocial Processes and Health: A Reader.* Ed. Andrew Steptoe. Cambridge: Cambridge University Press, 1994.

Curtis, Andre L., Thelma Bethea, and Rita J. Valentino. "Sexually Dimorphic Responses of the Brain Norepinephrine System to Stress and CRH. *Neuropsychopharmacology* 31 (2006): 544–54.

Cushing, B. S., and C. S. Carter. "Prior Exposure to Oxytocin Mimics the Effects of Social Contact and Facilitates Sexual Behavior in Females." in *Foundations in Social Neuroscience,* eds. John T. Cacioppo, et al. Cambridge, Mass.: Bradford Books, MIT Press, 2002: 901–8.

Daese, Andrea, Carmine M. Pariate, Avshalom Caspi, Alan Taylor, and Richi Paulton. "Childhood Maltreatment Predicts Adult Inflammation in a Life Course Study." Proceedings of the National Academy of Sciences (2007), 104, 1319–24.

Damasio, Antonio. *The Feeling of What Happens: Body and Emotion in the Making of Conciousness.* New York: Harcourt, 1999.

Dhabhar, Firdaus S., Andrew H. Miller, Bruce S. McEwen, and Robert L. Spencer. "Effects of Stress and Immune Cell Distribution: Dynamics and Hormonal Mechanisms." *Journal of Immunology* vol. 154, issue 5 (1995): 5511–27.

———, Andrew H. Miller, Maria Stein, Bruce S. McEwen, and Robert L. Spencer. "Diurnal and Acute Stress—Induced Changes in

Distribution of Peripheral Blood Leukocyte Subpopulations." *Brain Behavior and Immunity* 8 (1994): 66–75.

Andrew H. Miller, Bruce S. McEwen, and Robert Spencer. "Stress Induced Changes in Blood Leukocyte Distribution." *The Journal of Immunology* vol. 157, Is 4 (1996): 1638–44.

Doidge, Norman, MD. *The Brain that Changes Itself: Stories of Personal Triumph from the Frontiers of Brain Science.* New York: Penguin, 2007.

Dunbar, Robin I. "The Social Brain Hypothesis." In *Foundations in Social Neuroscience* op. cit.: 69–84.

Ells, Bruce J., Jenee James Jackson, and W. Thomas Boyce. "The Stress Response Systems: Universal and Adaptive Individual Differences." *Developmental Review* 26, 2 June 2006, 175–212.

Farooqi, I. S., and S. O'Rahilly. "Genetic Factors in Human Obesity." *Obesity Reviews* 8 (suppl. 1) (2007): 27–40.

Ferin, Michael. "Stress and the Reproductive Cycle." *The Journal of Clinical Endocrinology and Metabolism.* 84, no. 6 (1999): 1768–74.

Fox, Nathan A., and Stephen W. Porges. "The Relation between Neonatal Heart Period Patterns and Developmental Outcome." *Child Development* 56 (1985): 28–37.

Friedman, Elliot M., Mary S. Hayman, Gayle D. Love, Heather L. Urry, Melissa A. Rosenkranz, Richard J. Davidson, Burton H. Singer, and Carol D. Ryff. "Social Relationships, Sleep Quality, and Interleukin-6 in Aging Women." *Proceedings of the National Academy of Sciences* 102, no. 51 (December 20, 2005): 1875–62.

Fries, Eva, Judith Hesse, Julianne Hellhammer, and Dirk Hellhammer. "A New View on Hypocortisolism." *Psychoneuroendocrinology* 30 (2005): 1010–16.

Galon, Jerome, Deni Franchimont, Naoki Hiroi, Gregory Frey, Antje Boettner, John J. O'Shea, George P. Chrousos, and Stefan R. Bornstein. "Gene Profiling Reveals Unknown Enhancing and

Suppressive Actions of Glucocorticoids on Immune Cells." *The FASEB Journal* 16 (January 2002): 61–71.

Genazzani, Andrea Riccardo, Nicola Pluchino, Stefano Luisi, and Michele Luisi. "Estrogen, Cognition, and Female Aging." *Human Reproduction Update* 13, no. 2, 175–81.

Glaser, Ronald, Bruce Raabin, Margaret Chesney, Sheldon Cohen, and Benjamin Natelson. "Stress Induced Immunomodulation: Implications for Infectious Diseases." *JAMA* 281, no. 24 (June 23, 1999): 2268–70.

Gold, P. W., and G. P. Chrousos. "Organization of the Stress System and Its Dysregulation in Melancholic and Atypical Depression: High vs. Low CRH/NE States." *Molecular Psychiatry* 7 (2002): 254–75.

Greenberg, Neil, James A. Carr, and Cliff H. Summers. "Causes and Consequences of Stress." *Integrative and Comparative Biology* 42 (2002): 508–16.

Greenstein, Ben, and Diane Wood. *The Endocrine System at a Glance*, second edition. Malden, MA.: Blackwell Publishing 2006, 2008.

Hawkins, Brian T., and Thomas A. Davis. "The Blood Brain Barrier/ Neurovascular Unit in Health and Disease." *Pharmacological Review* 57 (2005): 173–85.

Heberlein, Andrea S., and Ralph Adolphus. "Neurobiology of Emotion Recognition: Current Evidence for Shared Substrates." In *Foundations of Social Neuroscience* (op. cit.): 31–55.

Hellhamer, J., E. Fries, O. W. Schweitsthal, W. Scholtz, and A. A. Stone, D. Hagemann. "Several Daily Measurements Are Necessary to Reliably Assess the Cortisol Rise after Awakening: State and Trait Components." *Psychoendocrinology* 32 (2007): 80–86.

Hellhammer, Dirk H., and Juliane Hellhammer. "Stress: The Brain-Body Connection." *Key Issues in Mental Health* 174. Basel, Switzerland: S. Karger, 2008.

Henry, James P. "Biological Basis of the Stress Response." *International*

*Physiological and Behavioral Science* 27, no. 1 (January–March 1992): 66–83.

Herbert, Tracy Bennett, PhD, and Sheldon Cohen, PhD. "Stressed Immunity in Humans: A Meta-Analytic Review." *Psychosomatic Medicine* 55 (1993): 364–79.

Jackson, Lisa R., Terry E. Robinson, and Jill B. Becker. "Sex Differences and Hormonal Influences on Acquisition of Cocaine Self-administration in Rats." *Neuropsychopharmacology* 32 (2006): 129–38.

Johnson, Elizabeth O., Themis C. Kanilaris, George R. Chrousos, and Philip W. Gold. "Mechanisms of Stress: A Dynamic Overview of Hormonal and Behavioral Homeostasis." *Neuroscience and Biobehavioral Review* 16 (1992): 115–30.

Kanakani, Akio, Nobukazu Okado, Kumiko Rokkaku, Kazufumi Hond, Shun Ishibushi, and Tatsushi Onaku. "Leptin Inhibits and Ghrelin Augments Hypothalamic Noradrenaline Release after Stress." *Stress* Sept. 11, 2008 (5): 363–69.

Kennedy, Adele, T. W. Gettys, P. Watson, P. Wallace, E. Ganaway, Q. Pan, and W. T. Garvey. "The Metabolic Significance of Leptin in Humans—Gender Based Differences in Relationship to Adiposity Insulin Sensitivity, and Energy Expenditure." *The Journal of Clinical Endocrinology and Metabolism* 82, no. 4: 1293–300.

Keysus, Christina, and Luciane Fadiga. "The Mirror Neuron System: New Frontiers." In *Foundations of Social Neuroscience* op cit.: 193–98.

Kirschbaum, Clemens, Stefan Wurst, and Dirk Hellhammer. "Consistent Sex Differences in Cortisol Responses to Psychological Stress." *Psychosomatic Medicine* 54 (1992): 648–57.

Klein, Stanley B., and John F. Kihstron. "On Bridging the Gap Between Social-Personality and Neuropsychology." In *Foundations in Social Neuroscience* op. cit.: 47–68.

Koolhaas, J. M. "Coping Style & Immunity in Animals: Making Sense of Individual Variation." *Brain Behavior and Immunity* 22 (2008): 662–67.

Krishnan, Vaishran, Ming-hu Han, and Eric J. Nestler. "Stress: Brain Yields Clues about Why Some Succumb While Others Prevail." *NIH News*, published online in *Cell*, Oct. 18, 2007.

Kudielka, Brigitte M., Angelika Buske-Kirschbaum, Dirk H. Hellhammer, and Clemens Kirschbaum. "Differential Heart Rate Reactivity and Recovery after Psychosocial Stress (Tsst) in Healthy Children, Younger Adults, and Elderly Adults: The Impact of Age and Gender." *The International Journal of Behavioral Medicine* 11, no. 2 (2004): 116–21.

Kudielka, Brigitte M., and Clemens Kirschbaum. "Sex Differences in HPA Axis Responses to Stress: A Review." *Biological Psychology* 69 (2005): 113–32.

Kumsta, Robert, Sonja Entringer, Jan. W. Koper, Elisabeth F. C. van Rossum, Dirk H. Hellhammer, and Stefan Wurst. "Sex Specific Associations between Common Glucocorticoid Receptor Gene Variants and HPA Axis Responses to Psycho-Social Stress." *Biological Psychiatry* 67 (2007): 863–69.

Landsberg, Lewis, and James B. Young. "The Role of the Sympathetic Nervous System and Catecholamines in the Regulation of Energy Metabolism." *The American Journal of Clinical Nutrition* 38 (December 1983): 1018–24.

Epel, E., R. Lapidus, B. McEwen, and K. Brownell. "Stress May Add Bite to Appetite in Women: A Laboratory Study of Stress-Induced Cortisol and Eating Behavior." *Psychoneuroendocrinology* (2001): 26, 37–49

Li, Linu, Jianmin Su, and Qifa Xie. "Differential Regulations of Key Signaling Molecules in Innate Immunity and Human Diseases." *Medical Library PO* (December 10, 2007): 174.

Liu, Dong, Josie Diorio, Beth Tannenbaum, Christian Caldji, Darlene Francis, Alison Freedman, Shakti Sharma, Deborah Peason, Paul M.

Plotskin, and Michael J. Meaney. "Maternal Care, Hippocampal Glucocorticoid Receptors and HPA Responses to Stress." In *Foundations in Neuroscience* op. cit.: 755–62.

Livine, Victoria, Miria Villegas, Carlos Martinez, and Bruce S. McEwen. "Repeated Stress Causes Reversible Impairments of Spatial Memory Performance." *Brain Research* 639 (1994): 167–70.

Loo, Ja Woo, and Ronald S. Duma. "IL—1 Beta Is an Essential Mediator of the Antineurogenic and Hedonic Effects of Stress." *PNAS* 105 no. 2 (1/15/08): 751–56.

Lupien, Sonia J., and Martin Lepage. "Stress Memory and the Hippocampus: Can't Live with It, Can't Live without It." *Behavioral Brain Research* 127, issue 102 (December 14, 2001): 137–58.

——, and Bruce S. McEwen, "The Acute Effects of Cortico-Steroids on Cognition: Integration of Animal and Human Model Studies." *Brain Research Reviews* 24, issue 1 (June 1995): 1–27.

——, Mony De Leon, Susan De Santi, Antonio Conuit, Chaim Tarshish, N. P. V. Nair, Mira Thakur, Bruce S. McEwen, Richard L. Hanger, and Michael J. Meaney. "Cortisol Levels During Human Aging Predict Hippocampal Atrophy and Memory Deficits." *Nature Neuroscience* 1 (1998): 69–73.

——, Alexandra Fiocco, Nathalie Wan, Francoise Maheu, Catherine Lord, Tania Schramek, Mai Thanh Tu. "Stress Hormones and Human Memory Function across the Lifespan." *Psychoneuroendocrinology* 30 (2005): 225–42.

Macky, Fabrienne, PhD. "Stress and Immunity: From Starving Cavemen to Stressed Out Scientists." In *Cerebrum-Ideas Brain Science*. Dana Press, Washington, DC (2008): 125–34.

Maier, Steven F., ed. Linda R. Watkins. "Cytokines for Psychologists: Implications for Understanding Behavior, Mood, and Cognition." In *Foundations in Social Neuroscience*. MIT Press, Cambridge, Mass. (2002): 1141–181.

Martinez, Manuel. "Biology and Therapy of Fibromyalgia Stress, Stress

Response System, and Fibromyalgia." *Arthritis Research Therapy* 9, issue 4 (2007): 216.

May, Eneran A., MD. "The Neurobiology of Stress and Emotions." UCLA Mind Body Collaborative Research Center. Winter 2001.

McEwen, Bruce. "Sex Differences in the Brain: The Estrogen Quandary." The Dana Foundation. www.dana.or/printerfriendly.aspx?id=4260.

———, and Dean Krahm. "The Response to Stress." http://www.the doctorwillseeyounow.com/articles/behavior/stress_3/index.shtml.

———, and Teresa Seeman. "Allostatic Load and Allostasis." August 1995: www.macses.ucsf.edu/research/Allostatic/notebook/allostatic .html.

———. "Estrogen Actions throughout the Brain." *Recent Progress in Hormone Research* 57 (2002): 357–84.

———. "Estrogens' Effects on the Brain: Multiple Sites and Molecular Mechanisms. *Journal of Applied Physiology* 91 (2001): 2785–2801.

———. "Physiology and Neurobiology of Stress and Adaptation: Central Role of the Brain." *Physiological Review* 87 (2007): 873–94.

———. "Protective and Damaging Effects of Mediators." *JAMA* vol. 338, 3 (1/15/1998): 171–79.

———, and Stephen E. Alves. "Estrogen Action in the CNS." *Endocrine Reviews* 20, no. 3 (1999): 279–307.

———, and Elizabeth Norton Lasley. "The End of Sex as We Know It." In *Cerebrum*, The Dana Forum on Brain Science 7, no. 4, Fall 2005.

———, Christine A. Biron, Kenneth W. Brunson, Karen Bulloch, William H. Chamters, Firdaus S. Dhabhar, Ronald H. Goldfarb, Richard P. Kitson, Andrew H. Miller, Robert L. Spencer, and Jay M. Weiss. "The Role of Adrenocorticoids as Modulaters of Immune Function in Health and Disease: Neural, Endocrine, and Immune Interactions." *Brain Research Review* 23 (1997): 79–133.

———, with Elizabeth Norton Lasly. *The End of Stress As We Know It.* Washington, DC: Joseph Henry Press, 2002.

————, Karen Bulloch, and Judith Stewart. "Parasympathetic Function." July 1999. http://www.macses.ucsf.edu/researchAllostatic/notebook/parasym.html.

Meczekkkalski, Blazej, and Alina Warenik-Szymankiewicz. "Hypothalamic Pituitary Regulation of Reproductive Functions." *Medical Science Monitor 5*, no. 6 (1999): 1268–79.

Millan, Mark J. "The Neurobiology and Control of Anxious States." *Progress in Neurobiology* 70 (2003): 83–244.

Need, J. Matthew. *How the Endocrine System Works*. Malden, MA: Blackwell Science, 2002.

Nelson, Rudy J., Gregory E. Demas, Sabra L. Klein, and Lane J. Kriegfeld. *Seasonal Patterns of Stress, Immune Function, and Disease*. Cambridge: Cambridge University Press, 2002.

Nepomnaschy, Pablo A., Eyal Sheiner, George Mastorakos, and Petra C. Ark. "Stress Immune Function, and Women's Reproduction." *Annals of New York Academy of Science* 1113 (2007): 350–64.

Norris, Catherine J., and John T. Cacioppi. "I Know How You Feel: Social and Emotional Information Processing in the Brain." In *Foundations in Social Neuroscience* op. cit.: 84–105.

Ochsman, Kevin N. "How Thinking Controls Feeling: A Social Cognitive Neuroscience Approach." In *Foundations in Social Neuroscience* op. cit.: 106–36.

Orrstein, Robert, and Richard F. Thompson. *The Amazing Brain*. Boston: Houghton Mifflin, 1984.

Pedgelf, David A., and Ronald Glase. "How Stress Influences the Immune Response." *Trends of Immunology* 24, no. 8 (2003): 444–48.

Playfour, J. H. L. *Immunology at a Glance,* ninth edition. Oxford: Wiley/Blackwell, John Wiley & Sons, Oxford, 2009.

Porges, Stephen W. "A Phylogenetic Journey through the Vague and Ambiguous Xth Cranial Nerve: A Comment on Contemporary Heart Rate Variability Research." *Biological Psychology* 74, no. 2 (February 2007): 301–7.

————. "Emotion: An Evolutionary By-Product of the Neural Regulation of the Autonomic Nervous System." In *The Integrative Neurobiology of Affiliation*, eds. C. S. Carter, B. Kirkpatrick, and I. I. Lederhendler. Cambridge, MA: MIT Press, 1999: 35–79.

Ratey, John J., MD. *A User's Guide to the Brain: Perception, Attention, and the Four Theaters of the Brain.* New York: Vintage, 2002.

Rohleder, Nicolas, Nicole C. Schommer, Dirk H. Hellhammer, Renate Engel, and Clemens Kirschbaum. "Sex Differences in Glucocorticoid Sensitivity of Pro-Inflammatory Cytokine Production after Psychosocial Stress. *Psychosomatic Medicine* 63 (2001): 966–72.

Roitt, Juan M., and Peter Delves. *Roitt's Essential Immunology*, tenth edition. Oxford: Blackwell Science, 2001.

Sapolsky, Robert M. *Why Zebras Don't Get Ulcers*, third edition. New York: An Owl Book, Henry Holt, 2004.

Schilbach, Leonhard, Wimon B. Eickhoff, Andreas Moziach, and Kai Vogeley. "What's in a Smile? Neural Correlates of Facial Embodiment During Social Interaction." In *Foundations of Social Neuroscience* op. cit.: 37–50.

Schonner, Nicole C., Dirk H. Hellhammer, and Clemens Kirschbaum. "Dissociation between Reactivity of the HPA Axis and the Sympathetic Adrenal Medullary System to Repeated Psychosocial Stress." *Psychosomatic Medicine* 65 (2003): 450–60.

Seeman, Mary V., MD. "Psychopathology in Women and Men: Focus on Female Hormones." *American Journal of Psychiatry* 154, no. 12 (December 1997).

Segerstran, Suzanne C., Shelley E. Taylor, Margaret E. Kemey, and John L. Fahey. "Optimism Is Associated with Mood, Coping and Immune Changes in Response to Stress." *Journal of Personality and Social Psychology* 74, no. 6 (1998): 1646–55.

Seyle, Hans. *The Stress of Life*. Revised edition. New York: McGraw Hill, 1956, 1976, 1984.

Sternberg, Estele M. "Neural Reduction of Innate Immunity: A

Coordinated Non-Specific Host Response to Pathogens." *National Review of Immunity*. Author ms available in *PNC*, January 25, 2007.

Taylor, Shelley E. "Tend and Befriend: Biobehavioral Bases of Affiliation under Stress." *Current Directions in Psychological Science* 15, no. 6 (2006): 273–76.

———, and Gian C. Gonzaga. "Affiliative Responses to Stress: A Social Neuroscience Model." In *Foundations of Social Neuroscience* op. cit.: 454–73.

———, Laura Cousins Klein, Brian P. Lewis, Tara L. Gruenwald, Regan A. R. Gurung, and John A. Updegraff. "Biobehavioral Responses to Stress in Females: Tend-and-Befriend, Not Fight-or-Flight." *Psychological Review*, 107, no. 13. (2000): 411–29.

———, Gian C. Conzaga, Laura Cousin Klein, Peifeng Hu, Gail A. Greendale, and Teresa E. Seeman. "Relation of Oxytocin to Psychological Stress Responses and HPA Axis Activity in Older Women." *Psychosomatic Medicine* 68 (2006): 238–45.

Tops, Mattie, Maarten A. S. Boksen, Albertus A. Wijers, Hiske van Duinen, Johan A. Den Boeer, Theo F. Meijman, and Jakob Korf. "The Psychobiology of Burnout: Are There Two Different Syndromes?" *Neuropsychobiology* 55 (2007): 143–50.

Wadhwa, Pathik D., Christine Dunkel-Schetter, Aleksandra Chicz-DeMet, Manuel Porto, and Curt A. Sandman. "Prenatal Psychosocial Factors and the Neuroendocrine Axis in Human Pregnancy." *Psychosomatic Medicine* 58 (1996): 432–46.

Wang, Jiongjiong, Marc Korczykowski, Hengyi Rao, Yong Fan, John Pluta, Ruben C. Gur, Bruce S. McEwen, and John A. Detre. "Gender Difference in Neural Response to Psychological Stress." *Social Cognitive and Affective Neuroscience* 2, no. 3 (2007): 227–35.

Weiss, Tamara, Kerry J. Ressler, D. Jeffrey Newport, Patricia Brennan, Alicia K. Smith, Rebekah Bradley, and Zachery N. Stowe. "The

Impact of Maternal Childhood Maltreatment on Obstetrical Outcome: Evidence of Early Transgenerational Effects." *American College of Neuropsychopharmacology Abstract* 13, 47th Annual Meeting, vol. 33, 12/2008.

Wust, Stefan, Elisabeth F. C. van Rossum, Ilona S. Federenko, Jan W. Kopper, Robert Kumsta, and Dirk H. Hellhammer. "Common Polymorphisms in the Glucocorticoid Receptor Gene Are Associated with Adrenocortical Responses to Psychosocial Stress." *The Journal of Clinical Endocrinology and Metabolism* 89, no. 2 (2004): 565–73.

Yun, Anthony J., and John D. Doux. "Stress Dysfunctions as a Unifying Paradigm for Illness: Repairing Relationships Instead of Individuals as a New Gateway for Medicine." *Medical Hypothesis* 68 (2007): 697–704.

## Chapter 5: The Foundations of Stress Relief

Antoijevic, Irine. "HPA Axis and Sleep: Identifying Subtypes of Major Depression." *Stress* 11, no. 1 (January 2008): 15–27.

Baria, Ana, and Phyllis C. Zee. "A Clinical Approach to Circadian Rhythm Sleep Disorders." *Sleep Medicine* 8 (2007): 566–77.

Barrenetxe, J. P., and J. A. Martinez Delagrange. "Physiological Metabolic Functions of Melatonin." *Journal of Physiology and Biochemistry* 60, no. 1 (2004): 61–72.

Basta, Marcia, MD, George P. Chouros, MD, Antonio-Vela Bueno, MD, and Alexandros N. Vgontzas, MD. "Chronic Insomnia and the Stress System." *Sleep Medicine Review* 2, no. 2 (June 2007): 279–91.

Benson, Herbert, MD with Miriam Z. Klipper. *The Relaxation Response.* New York: William Morrow: 1975. Revised foreword, 2000.

Buckley, Theresa M., and Alan F. Scatzberg. "Review on the Interactions of the HPA Axis Activity and Circadian Rhythm, Exemplary Sleep Disorders." *Journal of Clinical Endocrinology and Metabolism* 90, no. 5 (2005): 3106–14.

Duffy, Jeanne F., and Kenneth P. Wright, Jr. "Entrainment of Human

Circadian Rhythms." *Journal of Biological Rhythms* 20 (2005): 326–38.

Francis, Darlene, and Michael J. Meaney. "Maternal Care and the Development of Stress Responses." In *Foundations of Social Neuroscience* op. cit.: 763–74.

Greenberg, Jerrold S. *Comprehensive Stress Management*, fifth edition. New York: McGraw Hill, 2004.

Ko, Caroline H., and Joseph S. Takahashi. "Molecular Components of the Mammalian Circadian Rhythm." *Human Molecular Genetics* 15, Review Issue 2 (2006): R271–R277.

Lehrer, Paul M., Robert L. Woolfolk, and Wesley E. Sime. *Principles and Practice of Stress Management*, third edition. New York: Guilford Press, 2007.

McGrady, Angela. "Psychophysiological Mechanisms of Stress." *A Foundation for Stress Management Theories.*" In *Principles of Stress Management* op. cit.: 16–37.

Merrow, Martha, Kamel Spoelstra, and Jill Roenneberg. "The Circadian Cycle: Daily Rhythms from Behavior to Genes." First in the Cycles Review Series. *European Molecular Biology Organization Reports* 6, no. 10 (2005): 930–36.

Morin, Charles M., James P. Culbert, and Steven M. Schwartz. "Non-Pharmacological Interventions for Insomnia: A Meta-Analysis of Treatment Efficacy." *American Journal of Psychiatry* 151, no. 8 (1994): 1172–80.

Schible, Francis Levi-Veli. "Circadian Rhythms: Mechanisms and Therapeutic Implications." *Annual Review of Pharmacology and Toxicology* 47 (2007): 593–628.

Siegel, Jerome M. "The Reasons That We Sleep Are Gradually Becoming Less Enigmatic." *Scientific American*. November 2003: 92–97.

Smith, Jonathan C. "The Psychology of Relaxation." In *Principles and Practice of Stress Management*, third edition, edited by Paul M.

Lehner, Robert L. Woodfolk, Wesley E. Sine. New York: Guilford Press, 2007, 38–50.

———. *ABC Relaxation Therapy: An Evidence-Based Approach*. New York: Springer 2007.

———, ed. *Advances in ABC Relaxation Applications and Inventories*. New York: Springer, 2001.

Smith, Jonathan C. *Relaxation, Meditation, and Mindfulness: Essential Self-Training Guide*. Charlotte, NC: LuluPress, 2007. Retrieved September 2009.

Srinivasan, Venkataramanujan, Marcel Smits, Warren Spencer, Alan D. Lowe, Seithhikuprippa R. Pandi-Perumal, Barbara Parry, and Daniel P. Cardinalo. "Melatonin in Mood Disorders." *World Journal of Biological Psychiatry* 7, no. 3 (2006): 138–51.

Van Cauter, Eve, Ulf Holmbach, Kristen Knutson, Rachel LeProult, Annette Miller, Arlet Nedleltcheva, Silvana Pannain, Planaem Penev, Esra Rasali, and Karine Spiegel. "Impact of Sleep and Sleep Loss on Neuroendocrine and Metabolic Function." *Hormone Research* 67, supplement 1 (2007): 2–9.

Van Cauter, Eve, Karine Spiegel, Esra Tasali, and Leproult Rachel. "Metabolic Consequences of Sleep Loss." *Sleep Medicine* 9, supplement 1 (2008): 523–28.

Van Someren, E. J. W., and Rixt F. Riemensma-VanDerLek. "Live to the Rhythm, Slave to the Rhythm." *Sleep Medicine Review* 11, 2007: 465–84.

Wiebke Arlt, MD. "Junior Doctor's Working Hours and the Circadian Rhythm of Hormones. *Clinical Medicine Journal* (March/April 2006): 127–9.

Woolfolk, Robert L., Paul M. Lehrer, and Lesley A. Allen. "Conceptual Issues Underlying Stress Management." In *Principles and Practice of Stress Management* op. cit.: 3–16.

## Chapter 6: Nutrition

Adam, Tanja C., and Elissa S. Epel. "Stress, Eating, and the the Reward System." *Physiology and Behavior* 91, issue 4 (July 24, 2007): 449–58.

Akabas, Sharon R., and Karen R. Dolins. "Micronutritional Requirements of Physically Active Women: What Can We Learn from Iron?" *American Journal of Clinical Nutrition* 81 (supplement): 12465–515.

Angell-Anderson, E., S. Tretli, B. Jerknes, T. Foren, T. I. A. Sorensen, J. G. Eriksson, L. Rasame, and T. Grotmol. "The Association between Nutritional Conditions During World War II and Childhood Anthropometric Variables in the Nordic Countries." *Annals of Human Biology* 31, no. 3 (May–June 2004): 342–55.

Bourre, J. M. "Effects of Nutrients (in Food) on the Structure and Function of the Nervous System: Update on Dietary Requirements for Brain. Part 1: Micronutrients." *Journal of Nutrition, Health & Aging* 10 (November 5, 2006): 377–85.

Bourre, J. M. "Effects of Nutrients (in Food) on the Structure and Function of the Nervous System: Update On Dietary Requirements for Brain. Part 2: Macronutrients." *The Journal of Nutrition Health & Aging* 10 (November 5, 2006): 386–99.

Brummer, Robert J. "Nutritional Modulation of the Brain-Gut Axis." *Scandinavian Journal of Nutrition* 49, no. 3 (2005): 98–105.

Calder, Philip C., Samantha Kew. "The Immune System: A Target for Functional Foods." *British Journal of Nutrition* 88 (2002): 5165–76.

Challem, Jack, *Feed Your Genes Right*. Hoboken, NJ: Wiley, 2005.

———. *The Food-Mood Solution*. Hoboken, NJ: Wiley, 2007.

Chandra, Ranjit Kumar. "Nutrition and the Immune System." *Proceedings of the Nutrition Society* 52 (1993): 77–84.

Counsel, David, PhD. "Body Chemistry: Acid Alkaline Imbalance: The Root Cause of All Illness." *Wealth & Wellness*, October 17, 2003.

Cousens, Gabriel, MD. *Conscious Eating*. Berkeley, CA: North Atlantic Books, 2000.

Dinneen, S., A. Alzaid, J. Miles, and R. Rizza. "Metabolic Effects of the Normal Nocturnal Rise in Cortisol on Carbohydrate and Fat Metabolism," *AJP Endocrinology and Metabolism* 268 (1995): E 595–E 603.

Epel, Elissa, Rachel Lapidus, Bruce McEwen, and Kelly Brownell. "Stress May Add Bite to Appetite in Women: A Laboratory Study of Stress-Induced Cortisol and Eating Behavior." *Science Direct,* draft (November 3, 2000).

Esch, Tobias, Jae Wan Kim, and George B. Stefano. "Neurobiological Importance of Eating Healthy and Its Association with Pleasure." *Neuroendocrinology Letters* 27 (2006): 21–32.

Fernstrom, John D., and Madely H. Fernstrom, "Tyrosne, Phenylalanine, and Catecholamine Synthesis and Function in Brain." *Journal of Nutrition,* November 11, 2008.

"50/fifty Glycemic Food Index." http://www.lowglycemicdiet.com.

"Glycemic Index," www.cbn.com/health/nationalhealth/drsears_mind bodydiet.aspx and "Judging Supplement Quality," www.supplement quality.ram/z_askexpert/judging_quality.html.

Grimble, R. F. "Nutrition and Cytokine Action." *Nutrition Research Resources* 3 (1990): 193–210.

Hamer, Mark, Gail Owen, and Joris Kloek. "The Role of Functional Foods in the Psychobiology of Health and Disease." *Nutrition Research Reviews* 18 (2005): 77–88.

Herbert, Victor, MD, Subak-Sharpe, Genell J., *Total Nutrition: The Only Guide You'll Ever Need.* Mount Sinai School of Medicine. New York: St. Martin's Press, 1995.

Katz, David L., MD. "Do Diet Drinks Actually Cause Weight Gain." www.oprah.com/article/omagazine/20092_omag_katz-diet_drinks.

Klein, Johannes, Mathias Fasshauer, H. H. Klein, Manuel Benito, and C. Ronald Kahn. "Novel Adipocyte Lines from Brown Fat: A Model System for the Study of Differentiation, Energy, Metabolism, and Insulin Action." *BioEssays* 24: 382–88.

Leal, A.M.O., and A.C. Moreira. "Food and the Circadian Activity of the HPA Axis." *Brazilian Journal of Medicine and Biology* 30 (1997): 1391–1405.

Lopez-Varela S., M. Gonzalez-Gross, and A. Marcos. "Functional Foods and the Immune System: A Review." *European Journal of Clinical Nutrition* 56, supplement 3S (2002): 29–33.

Lovallo, William R., Noha H. Fara, Andrew S. Vincent, Terrie L. Thomas, Michael F. Wilson, "Cortisol Responses to Mental Stress, Exercise and Meals Following Caffeine Intake in Men and Women." *Pharmacological and Biochemical Behavior* 83, no. 3 (2006): 441–47.

Mazza, Mariana, Massimiliano Pomponi, Luigi Janiri, Pietro Bria, and Mazza Salvatore. "Omega-3 Fatty Acids and Anti-Oxidants in Neurological and Psychiatric Diseases: An Overview." *Progress Neuro-Psychopharmacology & Biological Psychiatry* 31, #1 (2006): 1–15.

Mendosa, David. "Revised International Table of Glycemic Index (GI) and Glycemic Load." www.mendosa.com/gilists.htm.

Morrison, Christopher P., PhD, Hans-Rudolf Berthoud, PhD. "Neurobiology of Nutrition and Obesity," *Nutrition Reviews* 65, no. 12 (2008): 512–32.

Moskowitz, D.S., Gilbert Picard, David C. Zuroff, Lawrence Annable, Simon N. Young, "The Effect of Tryptophan on Social Interaction in Everyday Life." *Neuropsychopharmacology* 25, no. 2 (2001): 277–89.

Neuhouser, Marian L., PhD, Sylvia Wassertheil-Smoller, PhD, Cynthia Thomson, PhD, RD, Aaron Aragaki, MS, Garnet L. Anderson, PhD, JoAnn E. Manson, MD, DrPH, Ruth E. Patterson, PhD, Thomas E. Rohad, MD, PhD, Linda van Horn, MD, PhD, James M. Shikany, DrPH, Asha Thomas, PhD, Andera LaCroix, PhD, and Ross L. Trentice, PhD. "Mulitvitamin Use and Risk of Cancer and Cardiovascular Disease in the Women's Health Initiative Cohorts." *Archives of Internal Medicine* 169, no. 3 (2009): 294–304

Nobre, Anna C., PhD, Anling Rao, PhD, Owen, Gail N., PhD. "L-theanine, a Natural Constituent in Tea, and Its Affect on Mental

State. *Asian Pacific Journal of Clinical Nutrition* 17, no. 51 (2008): 167–68.

Oliver, Georgia, Jane Wardle, E. Leigh Gibson. "Stress and Food Choice: A Laboratory Study." *Somatic Medicine* 62 (2000): 853–65.

Parker, Gordon, Isabelle Porter, and Heather Brotchie. "Mood State Effects of Chocolate." *Journal of Attention Disorders* vol. 92, issue 2, 2006.

Penev, Plamen, Karina Spiegel, Teresa Marcinkowski, and Eve Van Cauter. "Impact of Carbohydrate-Rich Meals on Plasma Epinephrine Levels: Cysregulation with Aging." *Journal of Clinical Endocrinology and Metabolism* 90, no. 11 (2005): 6198–6206.

Pick, Morcelle. "Reducing Inflammation, the Natural Approach." www .womentowomen.com/inflammation/naturalanti-inflammories.aspx ?id=1ampcamp.

Pitchford, Paul. *Healing with Whole Foods: Asian Traditions and Modern Nutrition*, third edition. Berkeley, CA: North Atlantic Books, 2002.

Pollan, Michael. *In Defense of Food: An Eater's Manifesto*. New York: Penguin, 2008.

———. *The Omnivore's Dilemma: A Natural History of Four Meals*. New York: Penguin, 2006.

Rogers, Peter J. "A Healthy Body a Healthy Mind: Long-Term Impact of Diet on Mood and Cognitive Function." *Proceedings of the Nutrition Society* 60 (2001): 135–43.

Rogers, Peter J., and Helen M. Lloyd. "Nutrition and Mental Performance." *Proceedings of the Nutrition Society* 53 (1994): 443–56.

Romero, Javier, Julia Warnberg, Sonia Gomez-Martinez, Esperanza Ligia Diaz, and Ascensia Marcos. "Neuroimmune Modulation by Nutrition in Stress Situations." *Neuroimmunology* 15 (2008): 165–67.

Sjostrad, Mikaeta, and Jan W. Eriksson. "Neuroendocrine Mechanisms in Insulin Resistance." *Molecular and Cellular Endocrinology* 297 (2009): 104–11.

Sommer, Elizabeth, MA, RD. *Food & Mood: The Complete Guide to*

*Eating Well and Feeling Your Best*, second edition. New York: Henry Holt, 1999.

Stanhope, Kimber L., and Peter J. Havel. "Fructose Consumption: Potential Mechanisms for Its Effects to Increase Visceral Adiposity and Induce Dyslipidemia and Insulin Resistance." *Current Opinions in Lipidology* 19 (2008): 16–24.

Takeda, Eiju, Junj Teraco, Yutaka Nakaya, Ken-ichi Miyamoton, Yoshinobu Baba, Hiroshi Chuman, Ryu Kaji, Tetsuro Ohmori, and Kazahito Rokuta. "Stress Control and Human Nutrition." *Journal of Medical Investigation* 51, August 2004: 139–45.

Tamashiro, Kellie L. K., Maria A. Hegman, and Randall R. Sakai. "Chronic Social Stress in a Changing Dietary Environment." *Physiology and Behavior* 89, no. 4 (2006): 536–42.

Taylor, Shelley E., Laura Cousino, Brian P. Lewis, Tara L. Gruenwald, Regan A. R. Gurung, and John A. Updegraff. "Biobehavioral Responses to Stress in Females: Tend and Befriend, Not Fight or Flight." *Psychological Review* 107, no. 3 (2000): 411–29.

Vasanti, Malik S., Matthias B. Schulze, and Frank B. Hu. "Intake of Sugar Sweetened Beverages and Weight Gain: A Systematic Review." *American Journal of Clinical Nutrition* 84 (2006): 274–88.

Vicennati, Valentina, Luana Ceroni, Lorenza Gagliardi, Allessandra Gambineri, and Renaldo Pasquali. "Response to the HPA Axis to High-Protein/Fat and High Carbohydrate Meals in Women with Different Obesity Phenotypes." *Journal of Clinical Endocrinology and Metabolism* 87 (no. 8): 3984–88.

Waladkhani, A.R., and J. Hellhammer. "Dietary Modification of Brain Function: Effects of Neuroendocrine and Psychological Determinants of Mental Health and Stress Related Disorders." *Advances in Clinical Chemistry* 45 (2008): 99–138.

Willett, Walter C., MD, with Patrick J. Slerrat. *Eat, Drink and Be Healthy: The Harvard Medical School Guide to Eating*. New York: Free Press, 2001.

Wilson, Paul. *Instant Calm: Over 100 Easy to Use Techniques for Relaxing Mind and Body.* New York: Plume, 1995.

Wurtman, R. J., and J. J. Wurtman. "Brain Serotonin Carbohydrate-Craving, Obesity and Depression." *Obesity Research* 4, supplement 4 (November 3, 1995): 4775–4805.

Wurtman, Richard J., Judith J. Wurtman, Meredith M. Regan, Rita H. Tsay, Jamie M. McDermott, Jeff J. Brue. "Effects of Normal Meals Rich in Carbohydrates and Proteins on Plasma Tryptophan and Tyrosine Ratios." *American Journal of Clinical Nutrition* 77 (2003): 128–32.

———, F. Larin, S. Mostafapoun, J. D. Fernstrom. "Brain Catechol Synthesis: Control by Brain Tyrosine Concentration." *Science* 185, no. 4146 (July 12, 1974): 183–84.

**Chapter 7: Exercise**

Aganoff, Julie A., and Gregory J. Boyle. "Aerobic Exercise, Mood States, and Menstrual Cycle Symptoms." Based on a paper presented at 28th Annual Conference of Australian Psychological Society, Bond University, 1994.

American College of Sports Medicine. *The American College of Sports Medicine Fitness Book*, third edition. Champaign, IL: Human Kinetics, 2003.

Andersson, Bjorn, Xuefan Xu, Mariell Rebuffe-Scrine, Kerstin Terning, Marcia Krotkiewski, Per Bjorntop. "The Effects of Exercise Training on Body Composition and Metabolism in Men and Women." *International Journal of Obesity* 15 (1991): 175–81.

Bergland, Christopher. *The Athlete's Way: Training Your Mind and Body to Experience the Joy of Exercise.* New York: St. Martin's Press, 2007.

Chatzi Theodoru, Dimitris, Kabitsis Chris, Malliou Paraskevi, Vassilis Mougios. "A Pilot Study of the Effects of High Intensity Aerobic Exercise versus Passive Interventions on Pain, Disability, Psychological Strain, and Serum Cortisol Concentrations in People with Chronic Low Back Pain." *Physical Therapy* 87, no. 3 (March 2007): 304–12.

Cox, Richard H., Tom R. Thomas, Pam S. Hinton, and Owen M. Donahue. "Effects of Acute Bouts of Aerobic Exercises of Varied Intensity on Subjective Mood Experiences in Women of Different Age Groups Across Time." *Journal of Sport Behavior* 24, issue 1 (March 2006): 40–55.

Crone, D., A. Smith, and B. Gough. "I Feel Totally at One, Totally Alive, And Totally Happy: A Psycho-Social Explanation of the Physical Activity and Mental Health Relationship." *Health Education Research* 20, no. 5 (2005): 600–11.

Dahm, Diane, MD, and Jay Smith, MD, editors-in-chief. *Mayo Clinic Fitness for Everybody.* Rochester, MN: Mayo Clinical Health Information, distributed by Kensington Publishing, 2005.

Dupree-Jones, Kim, and Sharon R. Clark. "Individualizing the Exercise Prescription for Persons with Fibromyalgia." *Rheumatic Disease Clinics of North America* 28 (2002): 419–38.

Editors of *Fitness* magazine, with Karen Andes. *The Complete Book of Fitness.* New York: Three Rivers Press, 1999.

Friedman, M. J. "Women, Exercise and Aging." *JAMA* 285, no. 11: (March 21, 2001): 1429–31.

Gleeson, Daniel, David L. Nieman, and Berte K. Pedersen. "Exercise, Nutrition of Immune Function." *Journal of Sports Sciences* 22, (January 2004): 115–25. www.optimalhealthconcepts.com/exercise stress.html

Jackson, Allen W., James R. Morrow, Jr., David W. Hill, and Rod K. Dishman. *Physical Activity for Health and Fitness*, updated edition. Champaign, IL: Human Kinetics, 2004.

Kanale, Jill A., Judy Y. Weltman, Karen S. Pieper, Arthur Weltman, and Mark Li Hartmen. "Cortisol and Growth Hormone Responses to Exercise at Different Times of Day." *Journal of Clinical Endocrinology and Metabolism* 86, no. 6 (2001): 281–88.

Leppamaki, Sami, Jari Haukkon, Jonko Lonnquist, and Tino Patonea. "Drop Out and Mood Improvement: A Randomized Controlled Trial with Light Exposure and Physical Exercise. *BMC Psychiatry* 4.22 (2004): 1–11.

Nabkasorn, Chanudda, Nobuyuki Miyai, Anek Sootmongkil, Suwanna Junpraset, Hiroichi Yamamoto, Mikio Arita, and Kazuhisa Miyashita. "Effects of Physical Exercise on Depression, Neuroendocrine Stress Hormones and Physiological Fitness in Adolescent Females with Depressive Symptoms." *European Journal of Public Health* 16, no. 2: 179–84.

Pedersen, Berte Klarlund, Heller Bruunsgaard, Marianne Jensen, Karen Krzywkowski, and Kenneth Ostrowski. "Exercise and Immune Function: Effect of Ageing and Nutrition." *Proceedings of the Nutrition Society* 58 (1999): 733–42.

Randolfi, Ernesto, PhD. "Exercise and Stress Management." www.optimalHealthconcepts.com/exercisestress.html.

Roth, David L., Ph D, and David S. Holmes, PhD. "Influence of Aerobic Exercise Training and Relaxation Training on Physical and Psychological Health Following Stressful Life Events." *Psychosomatic Medicine* 49 (1987): 355–65.

Sandoval, Darlene A., and Kathleen S. Mott. "Gender Differences in the Endocrine and Metabolic Responses to Hypoxic Exercise." *Journal of Applied Physiology* 92 (2002): 504–12.

Silver, Julie K., and Christopher M. Morin. *Understanding Fitness: How Exercise Fuels Health and Fights Disease.* Westport, CT: Praeger Publishers, 2008.

Teas, Jane, Thomas Hurley, Santosh Ghumare, and Kisito Ogoussan. "Walking Outside Improves Mood for Healthy Postmenopausal Women." *Clinical Medicine: Oncology* (2007): 35–43.

Transtadottir, Tinna, Pamela R. Bosch, and Kathleen S. Matt. "The HPA Axis Response to Stress in Women: Effects of Aging and Fitness." *Psychoneuroendocrinology* 30 (2005): 392–402.

———, Pamela R. Bosch, TimaSue Cantu, and Kathleen Matt. "HPA Axis Response Recovery from High Intensity Exercise in Women: Effects of

Aging on Fitness." *Journal of Clinical Endocrinology and Metabolism* 99, no. 7 (2004): 3248–54.

Tsatsoulis, Agathocles, and Stelios Fountoulakis. "The Protective Role of Exercise on Stress System Dysregulation and Comorbities." *Annals of New York Academy of Science* 1083 (2006): 196–213.

Wallman, Karen E., Alan R. Morton, Carmel Goodman, and Robert Grove. "Exercise Prescription for Individuals with Chronic Fatigue Syndrome." *Medical Journal of Australia* 183 (August 2005): 142–43.

**Chapter 8: Restoration: Techniques to De-stress**

Atsumi, Toshiko, and Keiichi Tonosaki. "Smelling Lavender and Rosemary Increases Free Radical Scavenging Activity and Decreases Cortisol Level in Saliva." *Psychiatry Research* 150 (2007): 89–96.

"Biofeedback: Using Your Mind to Improve Your Health." www.mayo clinic.com/print/biofeedback/SA00083/method=print.

Carrington, Patricia. "Modern Forms of Mantra Meditation." In *Principles and Practice of Stress Management* op. cit.: 363–92.

Chen, Keren. "Qigong Therapy for Stress Management." In *Principles and Practice of Stress Management* op. cit.: 428–48.

Cho, Yvonne, and Hector W. Tsang. "Biopsychosocial Effects of Qigong as a Mindful Exercise for People with Anxiety Disorders: A Special Review." *The Journal of Alternative and Complementary Medicine* 13, no. 8 (2007): 831–35.

Daakeman, Timothy P., MD. "Religion, Spirituality and the Practice of Medicine." *Journal American Board Family Practice* no. 5 (September/October 2004): 370–76.

Gay, Marie-Claire, Pierre Philippot, and Olivier Luminet. "Differential Effectiveness of Psychological Interventions for Reducing Osteoarthritis: A Comparison of Erikson Hypnosis and Jacobson Relaxation." *European Journal of Pain* 5 (2001): 1–17.

Ghoncheh, Shahyad, and Jonathan D. Smith. "Progressive Muscle

Relaxation, Yoga Stretching and ABC Relaxation Theory." *Journal of Clinical Psychology* 80, no. 1 (2004): 131–38.

Greenberg, Jerrold S. *Comprehensive Stress Management.* New York: McGraw-Hill, 2004. www.About.Com.

Klein, P. J., and W. D. Adams. "Comprehensive Therapeutic Benefits of Tai Chi: A Critical Review." *American Journal of Physical Medical Rehabilitation* 83 (2004): 735–45.

Koenig, Harold G., MD. "Religion, Spirituality and Medicine: How Are They Related and What Does It Mean?" *Mayo Clin Proc.* 76 (2001): 1189–91. Issue 12.

Koopman, Cheryl, Tasneem Ismailji, Danielle Holmes, Catherine C. Classen, Oxana Palesh, and Talor Wales. "The Effects of Expressive Writing on Pain, Depression and PTSD Symptoms in Survivors of Intimate Partner Violence." *Journal of Health Psychology* 10, no. 2 (2005): 211–21.

Kristeller, Jean L. "Mindfulness Meditation." In *Principles and Practice of Stress Management* op. cit.: 393–424.

Lee, M. S., M. H. Pittler, R. E. Taylor-Piliae, E. Ernst. "Tai Chi for Cardiovascular Disease and Its Risk Factors: A Systematic Review." *Journal of Hypertension* 25 (2007): 1974–77.

Lehrer, Paul M. "Biofeedback Training to Increase Heart Rate Variability." In *Principles and Practice of Stress Management* op. cit.: 227–48.

Lehrer, Paul M., Robert L. Woolfolk, and Wesley E. Sine. *Principles & Practice of Stress Management,* third edition. New York: Guilford Press, 2007.

Liden, Wolfgang. "Autogenic Method of J. H. Schultz." In *Principles and Practice of Stress Management* op. cit.: 151–71.

McGrady, Angela. "Psychophysiological Mechanisms of Stress: Foundation for Stress Management Therapies." In *Principles and Practice of Stress Management* op. cit.: 16–37.

McGuigan, F. J., and Paul M. Lehrer. "Progressive Relaxation Origins: Principles and Clinical Applications." In *Principles and Practice of Stress Management* op. cit.: 57–87.

Moraska, Albert, Robin A. Pollini, Karen Boulanger, Marissa Z. Brooks, and Lesley Teitlebaum. "Physiological Adjustments to Stress Measures Following Massage Therapy. A Review of the Literature." *ECAM* (2008) 1–10 doi: 10.10931/eca-/n—029.

Mueller, Paul S., MD, David J. Pleuck, MD, and Teresa A. Rummans, MD. "Religious Involvement, Spirituality and Medicine, Implications for the Clinical Practitioner." *Mayo Clinic Proceeding* 76 (2001): 1125–1235.

Norris, Patricia A., Steven L. Fahrion, and Leo O. Oikawa. "Autogenic Biofeedback Training in Psychophysiological Therapy and Stress Management." In *Principles and Practice of Stress Management* op. cit.: 175–208.

Rey, Oakly. "How the Mind Hurts and Heals the Body." *American Psychologist*, January 2004: 29–40.

Khalsa Sat Birs. "Yoga as a Therapeutic Intervention." In *Principles and Practice of Stress Management* op. cit.: 449–64.

Smith, Jonathan C. *ABC Relaxation Theory: An Evidence Based Approach*. New York: Springer, 1999.

———. "The Psychology of Relaxation." In *Principles and Practice of Stress Management* op. cit.: 38–56.

Taylor, Shelley E. "Tend and Befriend: Biobehavioral Bases of Affiliation under Stress." *Current Directions in Psychological Science* 15, no. 6: 273–77.

Turner, Rebecca A., Margaret Altemus, Denise N. Ypi, Eve Kupferman, Debora Fletcher, Alan Bostron, David M. Lyons, and Janet A. Amico. "Effects of Emotions on Oxytocin, Prolactin, and ACTH in Women." *Stress* 5, no. 4 (2002): 269–76.

Wolfgang, Linden. "Autogenic Training Method of J. H. Schultz," in *Principles and Practice of Stress Management* op. cit.: 151–71.

Woolfolk, Robert L., Paul M. Lehrer, and Lesley A. Allen. "Conceptual Issues Underlying Stress Management." In *Principles and Practice of Stress Management* op. cit.: 3–15.

## ACKNOWLEDGMENTS

Since we have written this book from the perspective of translating bench science to clinical practice, we would first like to acknowledge the brilliant, groundbreaking work of the scientists on which we have based our types and program. Every researcher and author listed in the Selected Sources has contributed to our understanding of the effects of stress on the body and shaped our recommendations about what works to counteract those responses. In particular, we would like to thank Juliane and Dirk Hellhamer, Bruce McEwen, Larry Cahill, Meier Stein, Doug Granger, and Nicole Gage who have been generous with their time and ideas.

Others have read our manuscript or inspired us, including Steven Kunkes, MD; Claudette Kunkes, PhD; and Alexis Johnson, PhD. Your professional takes and discussions have been helpful and encouraging. Barbara Garside, the librarian at Hoag Hospital, helped us immeasurably with our considerable research. Anna Miller and Rachel Miller worked from the East Coast to discover even more scientific papers. Susan Cohen gave us invaluable technical and emotional support.

Our office staff worked tirelessly and with good cheer even when we worked, at times without good cheer and humor, at our second full-time job during the last two years. We appreciate the support and encouragement of Susan Ermatinger, Rebecca Jansen, Raquel Richards, Cheyenne Chavez, Ashley Sylvan, Ana Alfaro, Brenda Cabrera, Annette Heath, and George Nichols.

This project was much more challenging and demanding than

we had originally envisioned. We followed our own advice and made sure we exercised and ate well. Natalie Sebag, Marta Cuervo-Ostrow, Adam Zickerman, and Dorota Knyswzewska kept us in shape and energized us.

David Vigliano, our literary agent, believed in us from the start. He found the perfect writer to help us shape the book we wanted to write as well as a distinguished publisher to guide us and to launch *The Ultimate Stress-Relief Plan for Women.*

We want to thank all the publishing luminaries at Free Press for their commitment to *The Ultimate Stress-Relief Plan for Women:* Martha Levin, Publisher, and Dominick Anfuso, Editor-in-Chief, thanks for recognizing that we had an important book to write; Leslie Meredith, our editor, and Leah Miller, assistant editor, for their exacting and tireless editing; Donna Loffredo, assistant editor, for her conscientious attention; Suzanne Donahue, Carisa Hays, Christine Donnelly, and the marketing, publicity, and sales people who strongly supported us from the start.

This book would not have been written without the vision and dedication of Diane Reverand, who was with us every step of the way. We also want to thank her husband, Sol V. Slotnik, for making us laugh and welcoming us to their home to process ideas and mountains of information that threatened to take over the entire house.

Our friends and families lived through a massive disruption in our lives for almost two years. For their patience and support, Beth thanks her parents, Max and Valerie Hampton, who were always interested in how the project was coming along and available to lend a helping hand. A special thanks to Jack and Mary Ann Hamilton for their continued love and support. She also thanks her dear friends Tiffanny Brosnan, Cammie Cassiano, and Susan and Robert Beall. Her husband, Jeff, and her sons, Jake and Asher, were ready with their ideas and tolerated her busy schedule with grace. Jeff always stepped right in and filled any gaps so that the project could succeed and their family life would not suffer. Their love and understanding was never more evident.

Stephanie would like to acknowledge her mother and father, Bee and Bud Nichols, for their lifelong influence and example of perseverance and hard work. Her three sisters, Paula, Lesley, and Beatrice, are strong and competent women, who have faced adversity in a way that inspires her. The entire Nichols and McClellan families have offered encouragement and support that was both needed and appreciated. Her sons, Michael, Tyler, and Gunnar, made sure she took some breaks for good meals, carved out time for family and fun, contributed to the research, and had endless conversations about the content of the book. Her life would be much less without her husband, Bob, who has always encouraged and supported her. He filled many roles during this process, including chef, host, computer tutor, and trusted confidant. He has dealt with the life of a man long married to a complex and passionate woman with style and assurance.

# INDEX

and inactive people, 182–85; incremental, 183; intense, 176, 181, 189–90, 242; and interval training, 187; keeping records of, 194; and lifestyle, 168, 182, 194–95; light, 189; moderate, 175–76, 182, 183, 189, 242; and mood, 176–78; as moving meditation, 172; and natural rhythms, 101; as natural tranquilizer, 170; and nutrition, 174; plan of action for, 190–92; Real Life about, 169, 180, 184; and relaxation/restoration, 177, 232; and rewards, 192, 193; scheduling, 192; skipping, 194–96; and sleep, 117, 118; and social networking, 191; sources for ideas about, 196; and strength training, 180–81, 187, 256; and Stress-Detox Program, 176, 192, 237–38, 242–43, 246, 250–53, 254, 256–57, 259, 261, 263, 264, 265; stretching, 251, 257, 261, 264, 265; and symptoms of stress, 3; thoughts about, 168, 195–96; tips for, 192–94; and type of stress response, 68, 72, 86, 196, 238, 242–43, 254; water-based, 181; and weight training, 242–43; and why exercise reduces stress, 170–71. *See also specific stress type*
expectations, 18, 20, 21–23, 24, 48
explanatory style, 21–23
Eyer, Joseph, 43

fairness fallacy, 24
fat: abdominal, 51–52, 172–75; and anatomy of stress, 46, 51–52; and apple and pear shape, 172–75; burning, 185; and exercise, 172–75, 179, 185, 186, 192; and glycemic index, 160, 163; and pH levels, 154; and Stress-Detox Program, 238; and type of stress response, 72, 238
fatigue: and autogenic training, 221, 224; and foundations of stress relief, 92; and glycemic index, 160; and nutrition, 123, 137, 144, 150; and pH levels, 153, 156; and relaxation, 96, 97; and sleep, 110, 113, 117; and Stress-Detox Program, 245; and symptoms of stress, 10; and type of stress response, 66, 75, 77, 78, 82, 85, 87, 245
fats (lipids), 72, 124, 128–29, 136, 139, 146, 147, 161, 166
fear: and ABC/ABCDE Models, 30, 31, 34, 35; and anatomy of stress, 46, 51, 53; and core beliefs, 25; of losing

control, 25; and psychology of stress, 18, 19, 20; and type of stress response, 72, 75
feelings. *See* emotions
fiber, 126, 146, 160, 161, 162, 249, 254
fight-or-flight response, 42, 43, 45–46, 47–48, 50, 54, 57, 58, 65, 68, 70, 95, 160, 171, 216, 242
fingerprint, 17
food: acid- and alkaline-forming, 155–56; anti-inflammatory, 166–67, 247, 249; circadian rhythm and, 102–3, 143–45; comfort, 146; functional, 122; functions of, 122; interactions of, 162–63; junk, 166; and knowing what and when to eat, 141, 143; labels on, 127; local, 130; log about, 126; and meditation, 208; organic, 127, 129, 130; prepackaged, 124; processed, 124, 125–26, 152, 162, 165, 166, 256; quality and quantity, 141, 143; whole, 124–26. *See also* nutrition
friendship, 56. *See also* tend-and befriend response
From the Bench: about antioxidants, 157; about Cycle of Renewal, 99; about emotions, 47; about exercise, 170; about friendship, 56; about history of stress, 42–43; about journaling, 233; about joy of napping, 108; about major life events, 177; about pessimism and health, 22; about PMS, 151; about sleep deprivation, 109; about socially determined emotions, 47; about stress-response, 64

gastrointestinal tract, 65, 73, 78, 82, 116, 117, 254–55
general adaptation syndrome, 43
genetics, 6, 15, 17, 44, 59, 61, 63, 114, 141, 161
ghrelin, 109, 149
glucose, 12, 70, 133, 134, 146, 160–63, 185, 186, 243
glycemic index, 160–63, 240, 248, 249, 256, 263, 264
God's Eye, 67
Goleman, Daniel, 17
green tea, 144, 150, 167, 239, 250, 256
guilt, 18, 19, 30, 34, 200

hair, 7–8, 10
headaches: and foundations of stress relief, 92; and glycemic index, 160; and nutrition, 134, 150; and

## ABOUT THE AUTHORS

Stephanie McClellan, MD, and Beth Hamilton, MD, both educated at USC, are partners in a thriving medical practice specializing in Obstetrics and Gynecology based in Newport Beach, California. As a team, they are affiliated with Hoag Memorial Presbeterian Hospital in Newport Beach. They have become widely known for their "outpatient hysterectomy" procedure, which is done with laparoscopy, almost no pain, little blood loss, and much faster recovery—two days to two weeks.

Additionally, Dr. McClellan has served as Chairman of the Ob/ Gyn Department and as a consultant to the hospital on women's health for ten years. She helped to coordinate the founding and building of their renowned Women's Health Pavilion. She helped raise an unprecedented $70 million for that project, and her vision shaped the highly regarded women's health center.